COVID-19:
THE FEAR AND POWER OF SCIENCE
Debunking the Pandemic

Joseph Lister

© Copyright 2020 - All rights reserved.

The content contained within this book may not be reproduced, duplicated or transmitted without direct written permission from the author or the publisher.

Under no circumstances will any blame or legal responsibility be held against the publisher, or author, for any damages, reparation, or monetary loss due to the information contained within this book, either directly or indirectly.

Legal Notice:

This book is copyright protected. It is only for personal use. You cannot amend, distribute, sell, use, quote or paraphrase any part, or the content within this book, without the consent of the author or publisher.

Disclaimer Notice:

Please note the information contained within this document is for educational and entertainment purposes only. All effort has been executed to present accurate, up to date, reliable, complete information. No warranties of any kind are declared or implied. Readers acknowledge that the author is not engaged in the rendering of legal, financial, medical or professional advice. The content within this book has been derived from various sources. Please consult a licensed professional before attempting any techniques outlined in this book.

By reading this document, the reader agrees that under no circumstances is the author responsible for any losses, direct or indirect, that are incurred as a result of the use of the information contained within this document, including, but not limited to, errors, omissions, or inaccuracies.

Table of Contents

Introduction 7
Chapter 1: What Is a Pandemic? 13
    Who Is Affected? 19
    The Reality 24
Chapter 2: How Do We Prevent It? 27
    The Four Acts Model 27
    The Guidance of History 31
Chapter 3: Bacteria and Viruses - What Are They? ... 41
Chapter 4: COVID-19 Facts and Figures 55
Chapter 5: The Science Behind Pandemics 73
    Biological Warfare 88
Chapter 6: Rise of Streaming & Gaming Services 91
    Benefits of Regular Video Game Play 99
Chapter 7: E-Commerce Boom 105
    Buy Now, Pay Later 107
    Why Switch to an Online Market? 111
Chapter 8: Electronic Payment Systems 123
    Fine Tune Your Business Model 133
Chapter 9: The Telecommunication Industry 137
    The Future of 5G 141
Chapter 10: What About Us? 153
    The Four Pillars 160
    Dealing with Emotions 166

Conclusion 175
References.. 179
Image References..187

Introduction

For everyone in the past year, COVID-19 has become a buzzword of massive proportions. With this comes fear, anxiety, and for some, a passive attitude. The reason there have been such varying degrees of emotions is mainly due to the depth and quality of news that is distributed to each country. The development of a pandemic, especially of this scale, has halted international and local travel while placing a large dent in most economies. Since February 2020, there has been a frenzy over the development of the first vaccine.

The presence of COVID-19 within the context of a pandemic can be easily explained. With the coronavirus having touched every corner of the planet, infecting those from all backgrounds, and even causing deaths, the category is fitting. The World Health Organization (WHO) first declared COVID-19 as a pandemic on March 11th, 2020. This disease does not discriminate or infect a singular group of individuals. It makes no difference if you are from India, Scotland, or Mars, you are at risk of becoming infected. No gender, racial, or social tier is immune against the coronavirus. However, what we do know is that socioeconomic status, living conditions, as well as population density, do play an important role in the rate at which this infection spreads. This will be discussed more in detail in the following chapters.

In this book, you will find a holistic approach to the COVID-19 discussion, where the main focus is to provide simple and easy to understand information so you can make more informed decisions regarding your health. You will find information about similar viruses and we will work to dispel some of the myths that have been making their rounds during this nerve-wracking time. These myths are at the center for individuals becoming anxious and depressed when emerging from lockdown. It is difficult for those who do not follow or have a natural affinity for scientific data, as the numbers that are being thrown around can be difficult to make sense of. I want to equip you with the methodologies that will enable you to understand the current climate of COVID-19 based on the most current statistics available.

There has been a large amount of research done on COVID-19 in the past year, especially on preventative mechanisms, the development of a vaccine, and how to ensure that people with preexisting conditions like diabetes and hypertension can decrease chances of contracting this disease. We need to regularly remind ourselves, "What about other people?" And this will definitely be answered here.

The pandemic has caused a huge strain on the livelihoods of many from different countries. To add insult to injury, the psychology associated with a pandemic leads many to stock up on essentials that they do not immediately need. What this does is skews survival towards those that are rich, leaving minimal resources available to those who are financially needy with limited accessibility. As a population, we tend to over-exaggerate the effects and needs during the time of a pandemic, because frankly, we have never had to live through one. This coupled with the conspiracy theories regarding how COVID-19 came to be, leaves minimal room for the facts about the virus.

In this book, we will talk about conspiracy theories with the main aim being to debunk them, try to remove any junk misinformation from your brain, and replace it with worthwhile and useful knowledge you can use to help others. I can assure you now that COVID did not start with someone eating a bat in China. As we take a step back and realize how the pandemic has affected every aspect of our lives, we are reminded how important it is to treasure the time we have in close proximity to others we care about. A positive thread that underpins the COVID-19 virus is that we are able to see the camaraderie within each small community, and our ability to help those in need.

Over and above looking at COVID-19 as a single entity, we are further reminded of the importance of remaining in a state of good health. The only way that we are going to successfully combat this pandemic is through stringent cleaning procedures (washing hands and sanitizing), social distancing to prevent spread, and a uniform mindset which keeps the future of the world as the goal in all decisions. We are all concerned regarding the impact this pandemic will have on our futures, both immediate and long-term; however, seeing as the world has survived its fair share of diseases with minimal resources, it is safe to say that we will also overcome COVID-19.

Chapter 1:
What Is a Pandemic?

Within the context of COVID-19, it is common to hear the word pandemic paired with it. For those outside the medical field, there may be some anxiety directly associated with the words used to identify infection patterns. This is why you need to know what it means when someone mentions this term, especially if you expect to really understand COVID-19.

In order for us to effectively analyze and establish the extent to which a pandemic affects the population, we need to define and differentiate the terms most commonly used.

- Endemic: When we look at a particular disease or illness that is found within a specific population, city or rural, we refer to it as an endemic. For example, chickenpox is known to affect mainly school-age children.

- Outbreak: An endemic that has grown substantially, to the extent that the estimated availability of resources is exceeded, will be termed an outbreak. It is important to realize that a disease diagnosis previously thought to be eradicated can also be referred to as an outbreak. If an outbreak is not controlled, it can progress to an epidemic and then further into a pandemic.
- Epidemic: A disease that affects a large number of individuals. These individuals are typically localized to a community that are established as a specific population group, or exist in a particular region.
- Pandemic: Contains the definition of an epidemic; however, this is seen on a global scale. A pandemic scale is achieved when a disease spreads over a multitude of countries and is not bound by borders.

When we relate the above definitions to that of COVID-19, we are able to see why it is classified as a pandemic. Initially, COVID-19 was endemic to

China, more specifically that of the Wuhan province in December of 2019. However, with it being transmitted by means of airborne respiratory droplets, those traveling internationally were unknowingly spreading the infection to people from other countries around the world. It was when cases of COVID-19 started to increase worldwide, coupled with the severe symptoms that it produced and in some cases death, that the World Health Organization (WHO) declared this disease to be a global health crisis.

Before we knew it, the virus had spread far beyond China, traversing the borders of foreign countries, and overseas that separate continents. It began infiltrating workplaces, grade schools and universities, and even halted regular social gatherings. We found ourselves adapting, finding methods better suited to the 'new normal,' and incorporating it into our lives. For instance, avid gym-goers found themselves improvising new ways to stay fit at home. Large plastic refillable water bottles became weights, and many backyards turned into running tracks. Life as we knew it had changed. However, that is the beauty of the human race, as we share adaptability to overcome a common threat despite rising difficulties that may further expose them to harm. We have come so far, and there is no backing down now.

What makes a pandemic interesting is the approach that different countries have to contain the spread and minimize deaths associated with the infection. Although the WHO provided general measures, which included hand hygiene, requiring healthcare workers to wear personal protective equipment (PPE), maintaining social distancing, and wearing masks, many countries around the world enforced more stringent measures. With countries locking down their population, imposing curfews, as well as halting all international (and some domestic) travel in an attempt to contain any further spreading within their borders.

It was through these strict measures that we discovered many individuals could be infected with COVID-19 and not show symptoms. This resulted in individuals spreading the virus unknowingly, and establishing the idea of 'herd immunity' within a population group. Herd immunity is what we typically find as time progresses within a pandemic. What it refers to, is a form of indirect protection due to a sufficient number of individuals developing immunity to a disease from previous infection. What this does is decrease the likelihood of infecting those with weaker immune systems, primarily due to less active cases. This is why health officials encourage those with weak immune systems to remain at home under strict quarantine until the infection rate dips back down. Those a part of herd immunity are no longer able to transmit the disease, and essentially the chain of infection is disrupted.

We need to remember that there is a fair amount of science involved when it comes to successfully monitoring the progression of a pandemic, as well as ensuring that it remains contained. Some of the effects of scientific discovery within a pandemic place a refined focus on response strategies. This means that research directly related to the cause of the pandemic needs to occur. An example where science enhanced preparedness for a pandemic is the Swine Flu/Influenza A (H1N1) pandemic that happened in 2009. Experts were able to predict the severity of the disease across many different population groups, which proved useful when field investigators needed guidance regarding the use of antivirals, and during the development of a vaccine.

What we did not expect to see, was the impact that science had on communication. Communicating valuable evidence such as that of evolving evidence of the H1N1 virus allowed the brainstorming of social distancing practices that would ultimately prevent spread. The same approach was undertaken when the COVID-19 pandemic surfaced. Science was able to surface the potholes in treatment modalities, which established a shift in focus towards finding a vaccine. If science was not involved in this process, time (an important factor during a pandemic) would be lost trying to decipher if a current treatment was successful. Science saves us time, and time saved can result in someone keeping their life.

Who Is Affected?

The question now is, "Who is affected by a pandemic?" The answer to this is as broad as the question, primarily because different individuals are affected in such a wide variety of different ways. To establish some relatability, we are going to look at how the COVID-19 pandemic has affected the world's population. Looking at healthcare professionals, what we notice is that they are not only tired physically but emotionally. A pandemic, especially one like COVID-19, has been mentally taxing on all healthcare professionals. The extra effort needed to correctly wear and change PPE, the mental stress of filling hospitals, and extra bodies needing care without additional staff available are just a few of the reasons why we are still dealing with this outbreak. Many healthcare professionals have put service before family, securing alternative accommodation for themselves or their family to ensure the virus does not spread to them, should they contract it in the field.

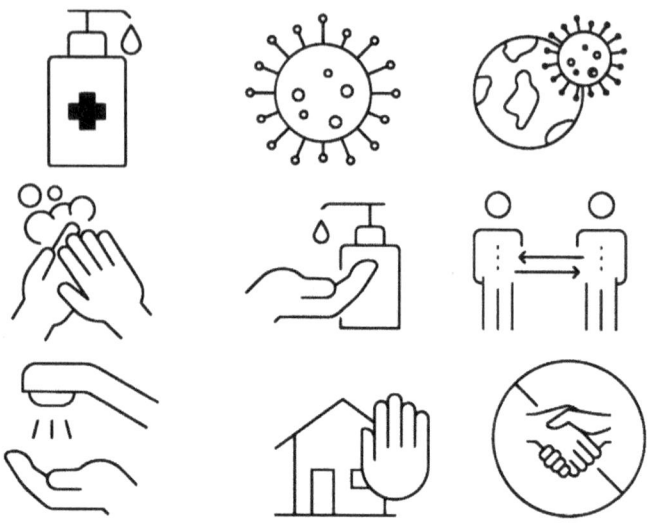

Small business owners have had to deal with federally imposed levels of lockdown that resulted in many closures throughout each community. With bills and rent still needing to be paid during the lockdown, the lack of cash flow caused expenses to outweigh profits forcing many to make the decision to give up. It's sad to see how this has impacted our society, but it is the reality that many have had to come to terms with. The impact on the economy has been a domino-effect, where businesses that close leave many individuals from all backgrounds and age groups unemployed. With many countries having a weak Gross Domestic Profit (GDP), low income areas have suffered, with many falling back into poverty they had only previously escaped. Mentally, business owners may have found themselves lost, developing depression, and even feeling completely hopeless. On the opposite end of the spectrum, many business owners have used this opportunity to define themselves as entrepreneurs, learning how best to navigate operations during a pandemic.

However, those that really suffered are the sick and elderly. The COVID-19 pandemic first presented itself as a flu-like virus, targeting the respiratory organs of the body. Studies surfaced detailing those with chronic conditions such as hypertension, diabetes, and chronic obstructive pulmonary disease would not only experience far more severe symptoms, but their chance of death due to COVID marginally increased. With that being said, when lockdown restrictions started to ease, and small gatherings started to take place as well as domestic travel, elderly individuals with chronic conditions were still advised to stay at home and isolate. We cannot begin to understand the impact that this has on their livelihood, and mental health. Not being able to socially interact with others becomes a struggle, especially for those who are close with their family, or require assistance from others.

Many parents were forced to adapt their work schedules to life at home, while managing their children's studies with most schools and universities closing after the initial stages of COVID-19. This proved to be especially problematic for those who did not have access to basic supplies normally provided by schools, computers, or reliable internet. However, a positive side of this issue was the compassion that many showed for those in their community. Individuals bought laptops and other school supplies for those in need. People put together food parcels for those with families that lost their jobs, many even offered their homes for people to quarantine.

This is where we get to the next generation of leaders having been affected, or the grade school children. One-on-one learning is what many find pivotal to learning new subjects, with very few individuals being able to effectively retain important information without direction. This has proven to be very difficult to adapt to, especially with the uncertainty of when school and universities would return to in-person learning. Those that enjoyed sports were cut off. Art and drama clubs disbanded, as they required in-person meetings to survive.

Taking a further look at university students, the integrity of some degrees were brought into question. The workload associated with a degree is a large one, with the want for a pass overruling the moral compass of most students. This has led to tests and exams being taken while notes are widely accessible and available to the students. However, universities have been aware of this and have put measures in place to curb this as much as possible. Some new testing options include making them shorter, providing a time limit for questions, as well as not giving the opportunity to go back to a previous question once completed.

The Reality

The COVID-19 pandemic has rattled our world, forcing us to embrace a new normal. Fortunately, despite the many negatives, just as many positives have arisen. However, the presence of effects as a function of time within and after a pandemic occurs needs to be understood. What is meant by this is the mindset and approach that individuals have to a pandemic while they are actively going through it and obtaining new information each day, compared to their mindset and approach to preventing the spread of the pandemic months after. What we are starting to notice, is a laxity in the stringency that people are adhering to social and personal protective measures as outlined by the WHO. Just because some believe that the worst part of the pandemic is over, they start to bend the rules to their own liking. Examples of how these rules are bent include not wearing masks in public, and not practicing adequate social distancing. It is the ignorance associated with these actions, that is inevitably prolonging the effect this pandemic is having on our lives.

COVID-19 is a formidable pandemic, and there should be no doubt as to whether it exists or not. The reality is, it is causing individuals to die, and fighting a pandemic is a collective effort. There is not one person that is excluded from being infected. With so many individuals being infected and showing absolutely no symptoms, the chances of becoming infected unknowingly, increase dramatically. This is why the entirety of the human race needs to come together in the face of this pandemic. It is real, and the only way we and our loved ones will make it.

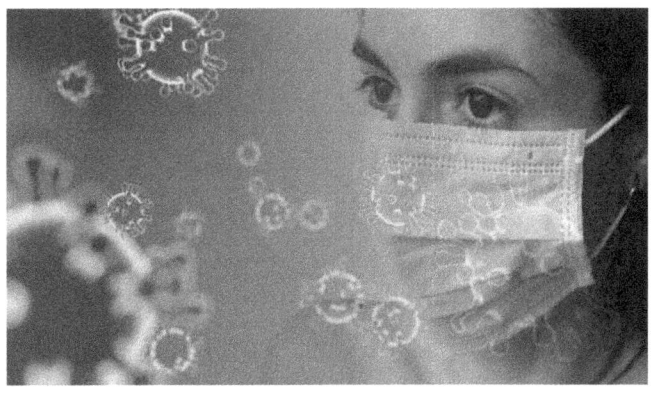

Chapter 2:
How Do We Prevent It?

The Four Acts Model

History has proven to be a very detailed source with how we manage pandemics. Now that you have developed a more sound understanding of a pandemic, the 'Four Acts Model' is important to take note of. A pandemic, as a social phenomena, has proven to produce drastic hardships and devastating after-effects. However, we don't need to look at COVID-19 to see this. A trip into history provides a look into the cholera pandemics that occurred in 1833, 1845, and 1866, respectively. It was by analyzing these outbreaks, a man by the name of Rosenberg, characterized the progression and unfolding of this pandemic, in a manner that constituted the four phases that provided a predictable course of a pandemic.

It is in the first phase, known as progressive revelation, that cases of a known disease start to increase rapidly. In this phase, deaths do not necessarily have to occur due to the disease; however, there is a strong chance that they can occur. The difficulty here is convincing other individuals that the region is on the brink of a pandemic. Many turn to conspiracy theories or skepticism when they hear talk of a pandemic, despite there being evidence of a contagious disease. While trying to prevent a pandemic, slow acknowledgement and acceptance by the population needs to be completely mitigated. A delayed course of action increases the risks associated with a contagion spreading. It is these key factors that form the pivotal role in these historical diseases. The problem with acknowledging a pandemic is you need to also realize the potential impact. This is why education is necessary to rapidly bridge the gap to acceptance; otherwise, the preventative phase will quickly become irrelevant.

Phase two focuses on 'managing randomness.' This means a system needs to be implemented that provides answers to arbitrary questions regarding the pandemic. By remaining are of the wide variety of individuals with different intellectual levels, we cannot expect a one-size-fits-all approach when relaying crucial information to the public. This dichotomy focuses on intrinsic or personal thoughts, as well as what external sources of information reveal about the virus. For example, many find that remaining steadfast in their religion and their right to practice it freely, predisposes them to comply with any new preventative measures. It is in this way, that preventing a pandemic needs to play to the strengths of a community when providing information. The importance of this cannot be overlooked, seeing as it is ultimately people that are responsible for mitigating the pandemic, or causing an increase in the amount of new cases. This is what happened with COVID; information was rapidly disseminated, which led to population groups feeling overwhelmed and anxious.

The third phase is 'negotiating public response.' This follows soundly as there is a shift from individual action to a collective effort. However, this collective action is done by the government agencies working to tackle the spread. This is where a further act to prevent pandemics comes in, the need for decisive leadership that is capable of containing and preventing the extent of positive infection cases reaching high numbers. Prevention cannot take place where crisis management is incoherent or incompetent. This is why leadership within a pandemic plays a key role. Through good leadership, you can reach the differing cultural values, economical, and social/political hierarchies that are present within each area. This remains imperative to successfully contain any contagion.

Finally, the fourth phase focuses on 'subsidence and retrospection.' It is at this phase that the existing responses to the looming pandemic are identified. These responses are then compared against a pandemic-preparedness plan that is constantly iterated. From this plan, public health management officials are called in to evaluate an area's response to the threat of a pandemic. This process is also an adaptable one, whereby current practices, as well as those that are yet to be performed, are evaluated to ensure that the pandemic's spread is halted, but also so that the interests of the people are taken into consideration. Other factors that are included for retrospective analysis, include that of the amount of susceptible individuals, deaths, as well as recoveries. The only way we can truly be prepared for a pandemic is by understanding its key features, as well as the practices implemented to successfully navigate a pandemic.

The Guidance of History

Although we have established that there is definitely a process that can be followed when a pandemic is evident, what we need to ascertain is the effectiveness of processes followed with previous pandemics and whether they would work in our current setting. One of the key factors is the change in accessibility to technology. When looking at the comparison between a cholera pandemic in the 1800s and comparing the level of technology that was present then, to what we currently have with COVID-19, they are almost incomparable.

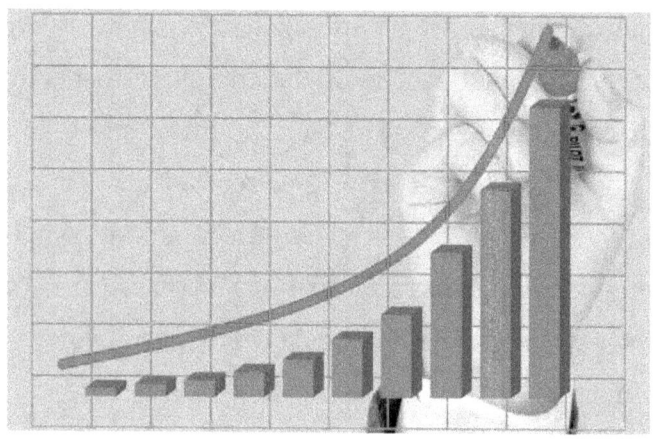

It is for this reason that we are going to delve into some of the most prominent and historically documented pandemics in human history. We will start with the Black Death, or bubonic plague which is one of the earliest documented pandemics. Having occurred in the mid-14th century, the area in which the Black Death was most prominent was across Europe, the Middle East, as well as northern parts of Africa. The degree of loss associated with this pandemic is very high, with a third of the population being wiped out in these areas. It is believed that the cause of this pandemic was the same bacteria that played an important role in the Justinianic plague.

Now remember, during this time there was no technology to breakdown or analyze DNA; however, we are now able to identify the spread across varying trade routes. This established the year at which the Black Death reached Italy in 1347. In those days, people believed that the plague was a product of rampant sin and the coming of an apocalypse. These forms of thoughts were not uncommon in this time period, especially seeing as a lot of the areas were Catholic. One aspect of the Black Death that differs from how we have handled COVID-19, is that in Europe, riots broke out as the population tried to make sense of the pandemic. This was particularly done through scapegoating outsiders, a factor that when mitigated can aid in the prevention of infections, as well as other external instances that hinder the quality of a human's life.

Similarly, in the second cholera outbreak in the early 19th century, riots also broke out. However, these reasons were primarily due to the resistance against interventions imposed by the state. Doctor's were attacked, especially because those with an infection feared their bodies would be dissected for medical research should they pass on. Luckily for people in this century, a deceased person's body is not allowed to be used for medical research without consent.

Cholera is a disease that is typically found in areas where there is limited to no access to clean water, thus it still exists to this day, just not to the same extent as a worldwide pandemic. We can thank our current technology for playing such a pivotal role in providing clean water systems worldwide. It is in this way that specific pandemics are almost completely suppressed. Technology is therefore a key component in the prevention of any pandemic. Another factor that is important in the prevention of a pandemic, and proven by cholera, is the trust that individuals need to have in leadership structures. In the 19th century, citizens had no trust for doctors or their government, making them rather reluctant in wanting to follow any sort of advice they offer.

The question then arises, "What can we do?" There is a wide variety of tasks from different domains that can be streamlined and better identified in order to prevent a future pandemic. A few examples of these are as follows:

- Transparency: Leadership structures, especially those in government, need to be fully transparent in the situation of an outbreak, and immediately if pandemic status has been reached. Trust is fostered through being honest with others, which is exactly what the government needs from its inhabitants for prevention to occur.
- Interaction with the public: Individuals in power, whether it be those that own businesses, or those that are making

decisions for a country, need to not only consult with specialists in the medical field, it also needs to consult with lay-individuals. It is not the specialists that will be as severely impacted by regulations imposed by the government (lockdowns, curfews, strict business capacities), it is the low to middle class individuals.

- Research: There is such a wide array of information available online, especially clinical research that can identify why some are worse than others. For many, there was no chance of a vaccine being developed. However, through identifying the possibility of novel infections, while still in the outbreak stage, the progression towards an endemic or pandemic can be halted. Where research plays a role is by being able to screen and identify individuals with the bacteria/virus, so that they can be isolated. The reason this is important has come through very nicely in the COVID-19 pandemic. Some individuals with COVID-19 did not show any signs of being sick, and were not told to isolate. These individuals were then able to walk around freely and infect others without knowing. If a tool to identify individuals with COVID-19 could be created through research, isolation would be streamlined, and the amount of cases would decrease dramatically.

- Infrastructure: There is an indication when a pandemic might strike, however, that does not mean we shouldn't be prepared. By pooling talent from both engineers and infrastructure specialists, we are able to create safehouses that will directly cater to the isolation of those infected. Furthermore, by equipping these safehouses with medical facilities, will ensure that the workload that is experienced within public hospitals is reduced, allowing healthcare professionals to still focus on their other patients that have not been infected.

The above four manners that aid in preventing a pandemic, cannot be performed as single entities, especially if full prevention is required. This is why pandemics also prove to show that approaches to them are a repetitive process. A problem that is faced is that these instances are not close together in time, which means that new generations who may have never lived through a pandemic, are now required to manage and prevent one. This is where documentation, medical or historical, needs to be taken with concise reports written and stored with head prevention specialists such as WHO. It is also difficult to say whether current measures will be useful in a future pandemic, as it is difficult to predict the severity of the next one. The next one could cause a mild flu, another could cause pneumonia, or infection, we won't know what the effects are until it presents itself.

However, what we can ensure is that the rapidity in response is heightened, as well as the flow of information within a specific region. This is why meetings that focus on pandemics, especially that of COVID-19, need to retrospectively analyze and iterate where general improvements could be made should we live through another pandemic. This is exactly where the people come into play, those below leadership positions. The role that we play is staying informed regarding the effects of widespread infections, planning ahead for when disaster strikes, as well as asking for aid when a struggle to maintain normal life is imminent. That is why asking questions and staying curious is so important. In the case of this pandemic, no question is to be ignored or thought of as irrelevant. That one question you may think is irrelevant, may be the one concern that that changes another person's life, if answered. If this concern is not addressed, the expectations set by governments for its citizens should not be expected to be followed.

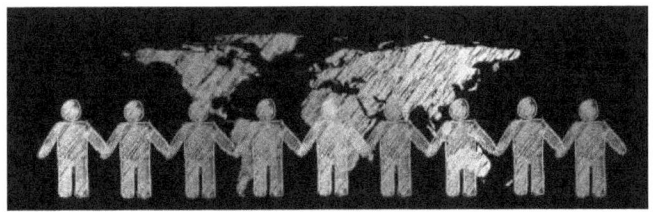

Chapter 3: Bacteria and Viruses - What Are They?

Bacteria and viruses are the causative agents when we talk about outbreaks, epidemics, and pandemics. However, the ratio of pandemics as a result is about equal, especially seeing as how they spread is completely different. In order to understand what causes a pandemic, one needs to have a clear understanding of the biology associated with a bacteria and a virus, as it is through this understanding that we can relate to modes of spread, as well as allow the indication of which treatment methods will be more useful.

Bacteria are a class of organisms that can only be seen under a microscope. They are composed of only one cell, which is why we term them as being a single-celled organism. It is this biological presentation that allows them to adapt and thrive in a variety of environments such as soil, ocean, and even inside the human gut. You may be wondering what bacteria is doing harm inside the gut, and you wouldn't expect this.

There are two different types of bacteria, simply categorized as good and bad bacteria. The bad bacteria are those that cause infections and illness, whereas good bacteria provide a large number of benefits for our body. An example of these benefits includes aiding in the absorption of nutrients in the gut while ensuring the acidity level is balanced. We also see good bacteria in food processing, where curdled milk is converted into yogurt or kefir, acting as a probiotic and supporting the digestion of food.

However, some bacteria have caused some serious effects on human health, to an extent of even being destructive. An example of this is MRSA (methicillin-resistant *Staphylococcus aureus*) that has been producing epidemic waves within specific population groups rather than a full-blown pandemic. Now with MRSA, it shows resistance to the treatment using antibiotics that would typically eradicate the bacteria *S.aureus*. By declining testing for MRSA, we allow the bacteria to grow and spread, leading to the possible development of pneumonia or skin infections. In severe situations, it can even be life-threatening.

There are even different shapes of bacteria, which allow us to see how they are transmitted, as well as how they attach onto surfaces when being spread. Round, cylindrical, spiral, and star-shaped most common appearances that we find with bacteria. These shapes present with different functions. For example, star-shaped bacteria are more likely to stick together based on the edges that exist, whereas the circular type can shrink when needing to travel through small openings.

When we start to take a look at how somebody gets sick from a bacterial infection, we need to remember that bacteria multiply. But how do they do that? A quick biology lesson tells us through a process known as 'binary fission.' It is in this process that the DNA (the disease-causing segment) of the bacteria is doubled, followed by a splitting of the cell into two identical cells. There are, however, other forms of reproduction that are specific to certain bacteria. An example of this would be Cyanobacteria that use a process called 'budding.' This process involves new growths on the original bacterial cell, where the newly formed bacterial cells just break off from the growths present on the original bacterial cell.

We have established that bacteria can be both beneficial, as well as detrimental to your health and the health of others. However, the detrimental aspect of bacteria is noticed more when we refer to its antibiotic resistance potential. When healthcare professionals unnecessarily prescribe antibiotics, bacteria can develop a resistance, creating a type of superbug that is very difficult to treat. With the difficulty in treating these superbug bacteria being on the rise each year, and more preventable deaths occur.

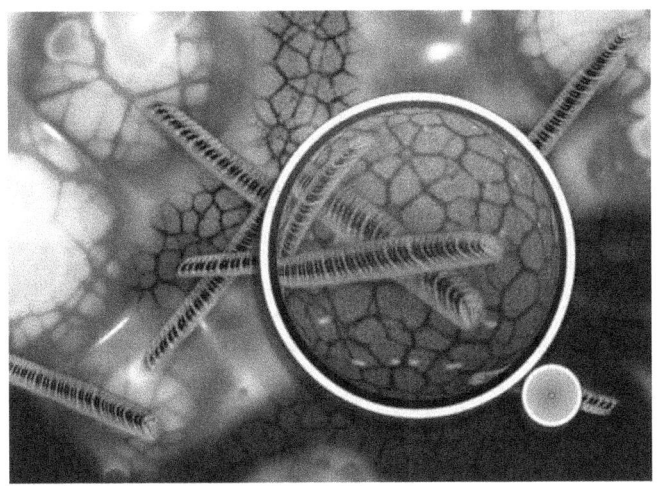

Viruses, on the other hand, are where we find COVID. To better understand the difference between bacteria and viruses, the biology needs to be dissected. Viruses are smaller particles than bacteria and do not have the ability to multiply when they are outside of the human body. Viruses are known to have caused some of the most well-known outbreaks, epidemics, and pandemics in history, including the Ebola virus outbreak in 2014, and the H1N1 Swine Flu virus that reached pandemic status in 2009.

Now that we know where they have been present in history, how did they get to that point? Viruses act by injecting their viral DNA (double-strand genetic material) or RNA (single-strand genetic material) into a human cell. These viruses detect a specific substance on the human cells, attracting them to the surface of the cell. Without this process, a human cell will not be infected with a virus. How these viruses come into contact with us while being inactive outside of the human body is typically through the saliva of insects or direct contact with fluids (if someone less than one meter away from you with a virus, was to sneeze without covering their mouth).

We can say that the DNA/RNA that is injected into the human cell, acts like an officer in an army. This officer gives instructions that ultimately result in proteins being formed that are viral and destroy human components. With this process we become ill. Although there are quite a few other intrinsic processes that happen, it is important to mention that it is at these intrinsic processes where the antiviral medication will act. It's important to note that antibiotics should not be given to someone with a viral infection, primarily because antibiotics aim for bacterial infections, not viral. It is the prescribing of antibiotics by healthcare practitioners, for viral infections, that are causing the high levels of viral resistance to medications.

When we compare how bacteria and viruses are transmitted, there are a few common differences present. Bacteria are typically highly contagious, especially in compact areas, because it is transferred person to person. There are quite a few other ways to transfer bacteria such as:

- When near a person or group. This can be anything from kissing to holding hands, and even standing shoulder to shoulder in a crowded space with poor ventilation.
- Coming in contact with the bodily fluids of an infected person. This includes genital fluids, and saliva spread through coughing and sneezing.
- Bacteria spreading to children in birth known as mother to child transmission.

- Coming in contact with bacteria on hard surfaces. Bacteria can survive outside of the body, this means that we are able to pick up bacteria by interacting with surfaces that have been contaminated such as doorknobs, toilet seats, or faucet handles then touching the face, nose, eyes, or mouth.
- Bacterial infections can also be obtained when consuming contaminated water or food.

With the above methods of transmission being similar to viruses, there needs to be a comparison where we can easily tell whether an infection is either due to a bacteria or a virus. Typically, an infection with symptoms that last longer than two weeks are likely due to bacteria. This is due to the rapidity at which the cells will divide in the body. With a viral infection, your symptoms don't usually get worse over time, which is the case with a bacterial infection. The reason that a virus won't get worse is the proteins that are produced in the human cell are exactly the same at all times. When checking for a fever, you will see a rise in temperature with a bacterial infection, not a viral infection. There is also a myth that if your mucus is green then you have a bacterial infection and require antibiotics. The reason this is false, is that the green color found in your mucus is actually due to substances that are released by your immune cells and in response to any foreign substance that enters the body. What this means is that you can get green mucus from a bacterial infection, viral infection, or just the seasons changing.

Healthcare professionals will typically take a sample of your blood, mucus or sputum, urine, skin, stool, or cerebral spinal fluid (CSF) if they cannot figure out whether your infection is due to a bacteria or virus and send it away for a wide range of intricate tests in a lab. This is considered 'culturing' for a bacteria or virus based on a human sample. These samples will typically be checked under a microscope by specialists who can discern your infection if there is one. They will also be able to tell you which type of bacteria or virus has caused the virus, making it that much easier to decide on the course of treatment.

Since COVID-19 is a virus, it is public knowledge that it is effectively transmitted through bodily fluids ejects by sneezing or coughing. However, there have also been investigations regarding how long it will stay on a specific surface. With it being able to only readily survive outside a human's body for a short period hand-washing stations have now been installed throughout all public domains, with proper sanitizing instructions in place.

Prevention and protecting from COVID-19, as well as from bacteria and viruses in general need to be adhered to. Specifically regarding COVID-19, we have seen by the increase in the number of infections what the repercussions are if protocols against COVID-19 are not followed. A few safety measures specifically tailored to the COVID-19 pandemic, are:

- Hand-washing is a preventative measure that removes a majority of bacteria and viruses when done properly. In terms of

COVID-19, it has been recommended to wash your hands with soap and water, and follow with an alcohol-based hand sanitizer.

- Social distancing has also been strictly enforced in most stores and social spaces, with stickers being placed on the floor at t one to two meters away from each other. Social distancing ensures there is no close contact between individuals and decreases the chances of spreading an infection.
- Wearing a mask when social distancing is not possible. It is recommended for you to wear a three ply mask to help reduce the spread of germs when in public spaces.
- Individuals subconsciously touch their eyes, nose and mouth throughout their day. However, remind yourself when touching items and surfaces that you do not know who touched that same surface before you. This is why it is important to never touch your eyes, mouth and nose, especially without washing your hands with soap and water first.

- Some habits that should be routinely acted upon include covering your nose and mouth when sneezing or coughing with your bent elbow. When you are not feeling well, call in sick, and do not go to work. If you find yourself with a fever, cough, or have difficulty breathing, make an appointment to see your doctor as soon as you can. If you feel sick it's important to limit all unnecessary contact with others.

We need to find ways to make the population see the validity and importance of taking these precautions seriously and act on them. The influence that the media has had on reporting false COVID-19 information has led to many not grasping the seriousness of what's happening. If we are able to implement the above precautions and show more individuals the benefits, the level of adopting these precautionary measures will likely increase.

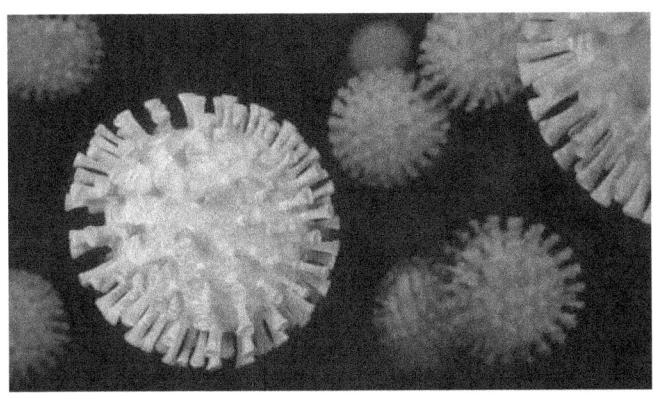

Chapter 4: COVID-19 Facts and Figures

COVID-19 facts are typically found lodged in between the false rumors and conspiracy theories. Luckily, if you know where to look, you are able to separate the lies from the truth. It is with this truth, that this chapter regarding all the facts of COVID-19. Viruses known as human coronaviruses, are relatively common interactions that we have on a daily basis. Mostly, these coronaviruses are found in animals, where only a very small percentage of them have the ability to cause diseases in humans. And COVID-19 triggerd by severe acute respiratory syndrome coronavirus 2 (SARS-CoV-2), primarily due to its effect on the lungs and nasal cavity.

COVID-19 has caused a surge in social stigma, especially to those of Asian descent. The reason for this stigma is due to the first cases of COVID-19 being identified at seafood and poultry markets in Wuhan, China. But, in order for us to understand the extent of the stigma, we need to know what this stigma encompasses. The social stigma associated with coronavirus is towards a group who share specific characteristics and disease. Typically, those that suffer from this are those that either have the disease, or those that remain in close contact with the diseased individual. Many of those that are labelled this way, may find themselves stereotyped and commonly discriminated against.

This treatment and regular isolation results in poor mental health. This knock-on effect extends further than just the person that is stigmatized, but also affects the caregivers, friends and family. With COVID-19, the stigma has been associated with three main factors:

- COVID-19 is a completely new disease, and coming from a well-known virus class, specifics regarding the SARS-CoV-2 strain have been hard to establish. This has led to a lot of unknowns being present, with heightened levels of testing and research needing to be performed.

- We are afraid of the unknown, and the extent of its capabilities, that we stigmatize those with the disease. Often, the reason for this is the individuals with the disease prefer to isolate themselves from the public who are so quick to judge. However, this method typically provides more harm than good in the long run.

- Fear associated with the unknown needs a physical representation to be justified, and this is why those that have the disease are labelled and discriminated against.

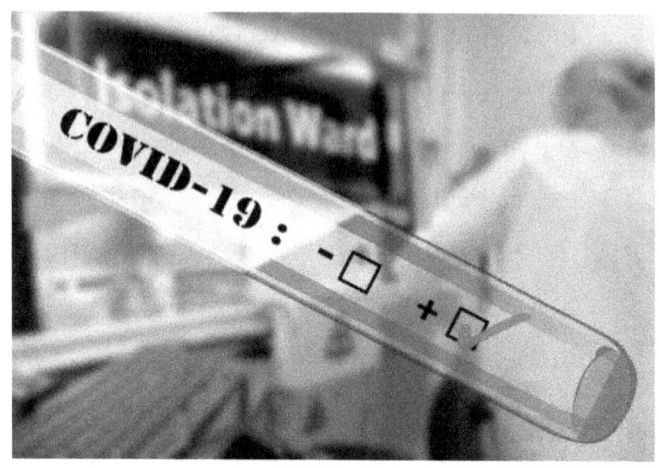

Now is the time to focus on the impact that a social stigma has on an individual. When establishing a stigma put on a person, the clustered mindset within the stigmatized individual will now function, and may contribute to one of two actions. These actions are whether an individual will cause the COVID-19 virus to spread more or remain dormant. Think of someone who has been told to quarantine because they have tested positive for the virus. The infected person has one or two ways they can respond. They may either think that they are above the virus and any stigma, not taking this information seriously so they continue to engage socially, ultimately spreading the virus. Alternatively, they might feel responsible for affecting the lives of others should they go outside, leading to the weight of the social stigma, eliciting a degree of isolation, which decreases the spread of the virus.

When one is stigmatized against, or when one begins to notice an apparent stigma, there are a multitude of responses that can occur.

- There is a strong chance that those that test positive for COVID-19 may be driven into hiding, by not letting anyone know that they are actually COVID-19 positive in order to avoid discrimination.
- The fear of telling others that they tested positive may result in them not seeking any form of immediate healthcare because of overcrowding, lack of medical coverage, or general fear of the process and treatment. All from what they've seen on the news, social media, or word of mouth from a distant source.

- The effect that stigmatization may have on another, is the realization that they are sick, which may result in a feeling of discouragement regarding the necessity to adopt healthy behaviors that promote a heightened immune system and improved quality of life. This is immensely important, especially for those that have tested positive for this disease.

Now that we have touched on the stigma regarding COVID-19, as well as some of the feelings associated with being stigmatized against, we should ask ourselves, "How do we address social stigma?" In order to address this stigma, we need to understand that stigma, as well as the fear of contracting a communicable disease, are real emotions. However, trust is seen as the core value necessary to combat stigma. Truth is usually practiced with a reliable healthcare team that demonstrates empathy towards those that are targeted. This is why it is of utmost importance to ensure that these measures are adopted, along with ensuring that effective physical practices are followed. What this does is provide a holistic approach towards managing a stigma, where those that are stigmatized against feel encouraged to not only keep others safe, but themselves too.

The need for communicating and supporting those with COVID-19 should not be overlooked. How can we expect individuals to take action against their illness if they continue to receive negative comments from others? This is why an environment needs to be created where open communication is established. This includes being able to converse about COVID-19 in a manner that promotes honesty. This is why we need to provide some tips to create this safe space for honest COVID-19 discussion.

It is important to realize, that even in the context of the COVID-19 pandemic, that words matter. If we are not careful in our word choice, especially when addressing someone who tests positive, there can be a perpetuation in the stereotypes and assumptions that are associated with being infected with COVID-19. What this further does is create a false association between the emotions that are felt towards COVID-19 (such as fear, anxiety, and depression), and the COVID-19 infection itself. Using the wrong word choice can keep people away from screening and testing centers, causing someone who is unknowingly infected but does not know it yet, and spread it. A few examples of proper word choice include:

- Refer to COVID-19 as the coronavirus, and not by the 'Wuhan Virus,' 'Chinese Virus,' or 'Asian flu.'
- Refer to those that have tested positive for COVID as 'people who have COVID-19' and not by 'cases' or 'victims.'
- When we speak about individuals who know they have COVID-19, we refer to them as having 'contracted' COVID-19, and not as someone that is 'infecting' others or 'spreading the virus.' The reason we avoid the latter is because it makes it seem that transmission of COVID-19 was intentional, which may even heighten the amount of reluctance present, especially regarding the

willingness to attend a screening clinic and possibly needing to enter into quarantine.

- When interacting with others, and the topic of COVID-19 appears in conversation, you are encouraged to speak positively about the situation and not just focus on the bad. By speaking positively, especially regarding prevention and treatment in place, you are instilling hope with others regarding this being an illness that can be overcome. This is done rather than instilling a sense of negativity within others, as they may have taken a hit to their mental health, making them feel hopeless and scared regardless of the outcome.

You may have seen that there is also a great emphasis on the public playing their part in the prevention and removal of COVID-19. However, the impact that specific individuals have on the positive outcome of COVID-19 should not be overlooked. For example, government officials, news reporters, as well as celebrities, have a very strong influence on the type of media that reaches the public. They themselves do not know the potential effects they have on not only providing accurate information but also in alleviating the stigma that has been associated with the Asian culture.

There is a strong focus on spreading facts regarding COVID-19. These are typically found on reliable health agency websites such as the World Health Organization (WHO) or Centers for Disease Control and Prevention (CDC). However, if there is not a strong focus on spreading true facts, a stigma can be overblown from the lack of accurate knowledge regarding COVID-19 transmission and treatment. Rather, a change needs to take place in our approach of spreading information regarding COVID-19.

This approach needs to focus on collecting accurate and truthful data, consolidating information, as well as disseminating what we know on a country by country basis. The reason it should be country specific is because the lockdown mandates, infection rates, and hospital sizes differ in each government. There also needs to be very specific information provided regarding groups vulnerable to COVID-19. It is also good to avoid using too much medical jargon, so information can be easily shared by word of mouth or online since many rely on these platforms to receive news.

We tend to forget the impact that social media influencers and leaders have on the degree of truthful information concerning COVID-19 is shared, as well as if people follow prevention and protection measures. Religious leaders play an important role in managing stigma, when you have these respected individuals speaking out against stigma, there is a higher chance the stigma will decrease, as opposed to individuals posting on Facebook about it. The information that these social influencers disseminate should be well-targeted, while remaining geographically and culturally appropriate. An example of how this can be done would be a city mayor posting a picture of them shaking hands with a leader from a local Chinese community on their personal social media account.

The voices of those who have experienced COVID-19 and recovered, need to be amplified. This means that stories and images of local people, as well as those that have supported them through their recovery, should be highlighted. A way in which this can be done is by implementing a type of 'hero' campaign where the caretakers and healthcare workers involved are honored. The role of this is to show the importance of specific individuals within the COVID-19 response team, but to also engage communities that have these individuals, to reduce the stigma associated with coming into contact with COVID-19. This contact can include willingly placing yourself in public or those that work in healthcare. It is important that when those in the hero campaign are shared that different ethnic groups are represented so it will reach a broader audience and decrease the stigma around the virus.

A very important concept that can be employed within the COVID-19, especially when sharing facts and figures, falls under the concept of 'ethical journalism.' What this refers to is the manner in which COVID-19 information is relayed to the public. For instance, if a reporter was to focus solely on the behavior of individuals who have tested positive for COVID-19, it would make these people feel they are personally responsible for it continuing to spread. Not only does this increase the stigma associated with those infected, but it may also result in heightened anxiety and further isolation.

There needs to be special care taken when reporting information on the effort to create a COVID-19 vaccine. This is because the sudden influx of news regarding vaccines can result in a heightened sense of fear, primarily as many may view that without a vaccine, we are powerless against COVID-19. It is better to focus on information that we know is true, and that has been shown to exhibit positive results when tested. Examples are prevention practices, how to monitor and treat symptoms of COVID-19, as well as when it is necessary to seek medical care.

There is an 'infodemic' of false information that seems to be making its way across the world faster than the amount of new COVID-19 diagnoses. What we need to do is not only oppose this movement, but establish a sense of collective solidarity that provides useful information.

the potential to support people and communities affected by COVID-19. Some of the manners in which this can be done are as follows:

- There is a wide array of misconceptions, rumors, and wrong information that directly contribute to the level of discrimination and stigma around COVID-19. This hampers the degree at which response efforts are successfully performed and can be avoided when primarily focusing on correcting misconceptions. Although this is important, to ensure these misconceptions are addressed, acknowledge people's feelings and behaviors in this state. We need to reassure those affected by COVID-19 that their feelings are valid. Furthermore, misinformation needs to be immediately halted, with a greater focus being made on the importance of preventing COVID-19.

- To prevent transmission, as well as to alleviate any of the concerns regarding COVID-19 experienced by a community, there needs to be a focus on collective solidarity. Typically, this is further enhanced through global cooperation. This means that sympathetic narratives should be shared in order to establish a humanized approach to COVID-19, as well as the struggles that it surfaces.
- A change in paradigm needs to occur from fear to facts. Ultimately, it is facts that are going to assist in stopping the spread of COVID-19, not fear. This means that not only should facts and accurate information be shared, but stereotypes and myths regarding COVID-19 and its effects, should be challenged.

COVID-19 is a real virus that did not appear due to someone eating a bat, or as a weapon of war in order to control the ever-rising population. How COVID-19 actually came to be is by the natural evolution of viruses. Typically, viruses change over time. What this means is that a virus that is common in an animal can undergo structural changes that allow it to be passed to a human. It is most likely that this is the direct mechanism of transmission that got COVID-19 to its current pandemic status. Although it is real, it is the job of the human race to aid in the abolishment of this virus.

The way we spread information and interact with those with COVID-19 will ultimately influence the length at which we will allow COVID-19 to alter the way we live our lives. We are our own barriers, and once we realize it, we can focus on creating a partnership with each other that focuses on the importance of human emotions and not putting individuals into a stigmatized box.

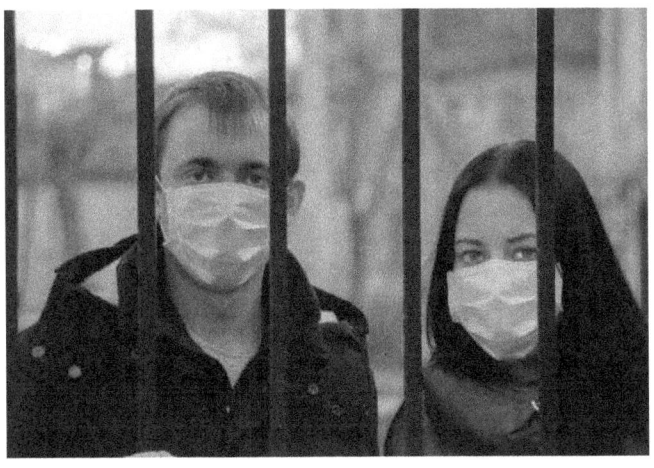

Chapter 5:
The Science Behind Pandemics

In a previous chapter, there was a brief explanation of the impact and role of science during a pandemic. Now we wanted to provide a bit more insight regarding where science fits in before, during, and after the pandemic. When we focus on the before, we see science providing a rather descriptive approach towards how this pandemic can play out. This primarily focuses on the use of statistics and previous data from other outbreaks to establish which type of response, as well as the severity. Furthermore, the use of science allows a comparison to evaluate longevity, severity and necessary resources. In terms of COVID-19, specific predictions have been made on the mortality rate, which informed the degree and type of preventative measures that should be taken.

How preventative measures were analyzed and instituted, has been based on the data collected from a variety of different pandemics, inputting this data to develop trends that define the risk that a pandemic has on the population. What the third edition of 'Disease Control Priorities' informs us of is that there is no 'one size fits all' approach when combatting a pandemic. Factors that include population growth, a heightened demand for animal protein, habitat loss, climate change and an increase in urbanization, are but a few factors that need to be considered when analyzing the likelihood of local pandemic infiltration, and the possible spread of the virus or bacteria. It was for this reason, coupled with the statistical estimation of the world's population reaching 9.7 billion by 2050, that social distancing and mask wearing practices were necessary.

One can even use the current data of COVID-19 to establish immediate future measures to combat its spread. This can be done by looking at the CDC library. In a bulletin posted on December 8th, 2020, reference was made to an increase in the prevalence of psychiatric disorders by 3% in patients with COVID-19. Further insights include that those diagnosed with a psychiatric condition within the last year were more likely to contract COVID-19 than those previously undiagnosed. What this means is that access to mental health services needs to be ingrained within the management of not only COVID-19, but also with people in general. If the declining states of mental health can be effectively halted, the degree of COVID-19 spread will follow suit.

During the pandemic, depending on the symptoms of the virus, research is required to understand the genetic makeup, how it makes a person sick, and how to cure them. This is when the big pharmaceutical companies begin to focus a majority of their resources on testing medication. We now see Russia, Great Britain, China, and South Africa making great strides in this race to get their first. In accordance with the Johns Hopkins Center for Health Security, 165 candidate vaccines for COVID-19 have been authorized in the United States of America since August 2020. When we take a look at the United Kingdom, as of early December 2020, their mass COVID-19 immunization program has begun, starting with the immunizations of the elderly. Pfizer has informed the public that their COVID-19 vaccine must be done in two doses for maximal immunity to be established. According to Pfizer, the United Kingdom has further ordered more than 40 million vaccines, to be administered in subsequent waves, for selected candidates. Pfizer says that the time gap between each dose needing to be administered is seven to ten days. A person who has complied with both doses within the given timeframe should then have an established immunity against COVID-19.

As of December 2020 there are four main vaccines that have entered into phase three clinical trials. To provide some more insight, these are how they compare with each other:

- Oxford University/AstraZeneca: This vaccine produced in the United Kingdom uses the COVID-19 virus, modifying it so that its vaccine counterpart can be created.

Having shown effectiveness of between 62% and 90% it remains the cheapest form of the COVID-19 vaccine at $4 per dose. With there being two doses required for a person to become immune, an added advantage is that this vaccine can be stored in a regular fridge (with a temperature of between 3°C and 5°C).

- Moderna: A vaccine that uses a specific part of genetic material known as RNA, modifying it to be effective against COVID-19 whilst not being rejected by the body's immune system. With an effectiveness of 95%, this two dose vaccine shows to be one of the most promising, along with its storage being up to six months in a temperature of -20°C. This vaccine is the most expensive, sitting at $33 per dose.

- Pfizer/BioNTech: A German and United States of America collaboration that, like the Moderna, focuses on modifying genetic RNA. However, where it differs is in the cost ($20 per dose), and its temperature requirements being -70°C. This vaccine needs two doses, and also has a 95% effectiveness score based on the preliminary phase three clinical trial results.

- Gamaleya (Sputnik V): A Russian produced vaccine that uses a viral vector, much like that of the Oxford/AstraZeneca vaccine, in order to impart its immunity to the human body. Also needing two doses for maximum immunity, it has a 92% effectiveness score, with its stability being its main benefit. This vaccine can be stored in a regular fridge, and is in a dry form that needs to be redistributed before administration. This vaccine will cost $10 per dose.

Although we are living in a pandemic, it is a rather exciting time for modern medicine, especially as vaccine results are showing great effectiveness. However, what many find rather confusing, is the question of who will be selected for the first few waves of the COVID-19 vaccine? The categories of individuals who will be a part of these initial vaccines, in accordance with the CDC, are the following:

- Healthcare workers: In order to ensure that the fight against COVID-19 remains strong, the front line workers need to be protected. This means that those that provide critical care to those that are infected with COVID-19, need to be protected in order to continue doing so. With healthcare workers who are COVID-19 positive (especially those that are showing no symptoms) being the main transmission avenue for patients within the healthcare facilities, the need for healthcare workers to be the first to get vaccinated is supported.
- Workers present in essential and critical industries: Individuals that are present in occupations that are a necessity for the economy to continue functioning, will also qualify to receive the vaccine. Not only will these individuals be required to work, however, many of their jobs (e.g military workers, grocery store workers) will require

interactions with the general public, increasing their risk for contracting COVID-19.

- Individuals with confirmed underlying medical conditions: Regardless of the age of these individuals, they are at an increased risk for presenting with severe COVID-19 symptoms. Providing these individuals (e.g those with hypertension, diabetes and respiratory illnesses) with early access to the vaccine will impart health and safety onto a group of individuals that have been disproportionately affected by COVID-19. It is most likely those that are older than 65 years of age that would fall into this category.

We see that science has impacted how we manage those infected by COVID-19. The manner in which we see this is in hospitals, and their use of ventilators. With the role of science needing to have acted with haste, the Imperial College of London in collaboration with King's College focused on the possibility of treating two patients who are COVID-19 positive using one ventilator. With there being recognized dangers of sharing a ventilator, through using variable resistances and one-way valves, two patients with lung problems requiring different rates and pressures of airflow, can be treated. With the science of medicine collaborating with biomedical engineering, the ability for ventilator splitting to occur can be achieved.

Science will also have a great impact at the end of the pandemic, as it will allow a more modernized approach to containing outbreaks. As each new virus occurs, the control and containment will be effectively altered. We are starting to readily see these future approaches being implemented when we look at the United Kingdom, as well as the Biden administration in the United States of America. With Trump's effort to withdraw from the World Health Organization, the U.S. government needed to take an innovative approach towards dealing with the pandemic. With COVID-19 numbers constantly on the rise in the United States of America, incoming president-elect Joe Biden has established meetings with stakeholders that are a part of the COVAX initiative for global distribution of the COVID-19 vaccine. BBC News has also confirmed that Joe Biden has committed to providing vaccines to 100 million Americans during his first 100 days in office. He further plans to strengthen mask mandates within the country, as well as categorizing getting kids back to school as a national priority.

It is within this context that the integration of politics with treatment decisions comes into play. When the ministers of countries are to enforce stringent social distancing protocols, they are doing so based on advice that has been supplied to them by scientific advisory committees. It is in this way that relying solely on science to influence policy is to misunderstand the core of what science is. When we take a look at two different countries, Hong Kong and New Zealand, we are able to see that their varying degrees of forcible lockdowns were based on political decisions informed by scientific findings, not by science itself. Transparency is key within the political realm, especially when there is a pandemic present. There needs to be policies that are created that benefit the public, not just those that are a quick fix with no scientific support for implementation.

Across the world, the governments of countries are further starting to make waves in the fight against COVID-19. The South African government has been rolled in the phase three vaccine trial piloted by Pfizer. The reason for this enrollment is based on the need for diversity amongst the trial population, seeing as South Africa has the most Human Immunodeficiency Virus (HIV) infections worldwide. Across the African continent, the vaccine produced by the collaborative efforts of Oxford University and AstraZeneca are beginning to be distributed via international airlines to African countries, although the exact locations have yet to be confirmed. With Ethiopian Air currently being in conversations with Shenzhen's health department, structured deliveries of essential medicines, including that of the manufactured COVID-19 vaccine, will be delivered to Addis Ababa two times per week. As the clinical data begins to surface regarding the effectiveness of the different vaccines available worldwide, clinical trials will be able to become more widespread.

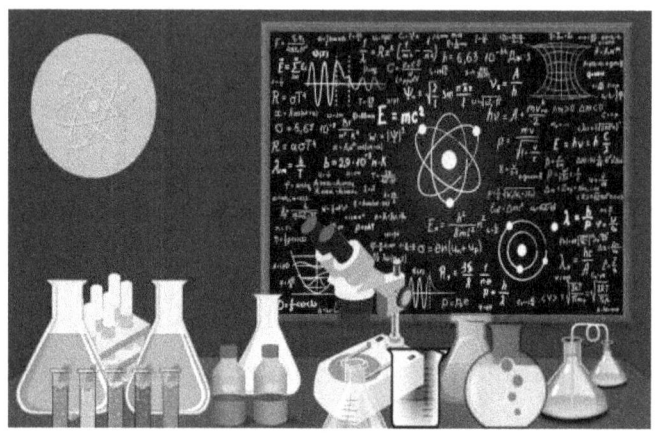

To see the importance of science in the context of COVID-19, we need to delve into what would have happened if we did not have any system to rely on.

Science plays an important role in allowing the public to come to terms with how a pandemic can influence their lives. Without research, many solutions to infectious disease outbreaks would not exist. Not only does this heighten the degree of fear and anxiety that is present, but it also results in individuals not understanding the necessity of preventative and protective measures being put in place. Ultimately, without science, the amount of infections would increase dramatically.

It also plays a role in identifying the most safe, effective and high quality treatment available for everyone regardless of age. It has played such a pivotal role in saving the lives of others, while establishing a practical way to handle an outbreak. If science was not present, there would most likely be no concept of treatment for COVID-19. Science further collates information to establish a final deduction. It is these deductions that inform protective mechanisms that prevent spread. An example of this is the science behind measuring the sizes of viruses and bacteria, impacting the best means to prevent COVID-19 spread when coughing. The British Medical Journal (BMJ) conducted a randomized control study that featured 1,067 healthcare workers. The cloth mask was compared with just using the elbow of one's arm when coughing into, as well as a combined effort of wearing both a mask and coughing into one's elbow. Wearing a mask, as well as coughing into your elbow, showed a 77% increase in localized coughing, preventing spread more than if one was to cough into one's elbow without having donned a cloth mask. With 97% of particles penetrating a cloth mask, and only 44% penetrating a medical-grade mask, based on the limited accessibility to the latter, cloth masks were used in this study.

Without scientific advancement, there would be no hope. This plays such an important role in ensuring that mental health remains intact. The manners in which this has occurred is through technological advancements of communication. Video calling and social media have had such a great influence on positive mental health, as it has prompted a sense of togetherness, even in times of isolation.

Now that we have established that scientific advancement is necessary, we can delve a bit deeper into which branches of science that can help with a pandemic. There are up to 20 basic branches of science, not including all of the hybrid fields that have popped up in modern times. You wouldn't think paleontology has anything to do with pandemic science. Well you are wrong, the study of ancient and geological periods can provide core information regarding virus and bacteria origins, as well as how they have the potential to cause a pandemic. Seeing as many viruses and bacteria can remain dormant within fossils, they can be excavated and studied.

Medicine and mycology are probably the most important branches of science in the context of a pandemic. The study of medicine deals with illness, disease, as well as the recovery and prevention of a specific disease. Medicine ties in with Mycology (the study of fungi), as it focuses on disease causing organisms. In terms of the COVID-19, our immune systems become weakened, increasing the chances of other infections to occur. Physiology, human biology, microbiology, genetics, and radiology also are called into play when researching COVID-19.

Biological Warfare

Biological warfare has become a conspiracy theory of great interest since the COVID-19 pandemic has taken over. This is defined as the use of a biological agent (virus, bacteria, fungus, parasite) to attack a group of people, also known as bioterrorism. It is through stories of bio-attacks, or 'germ warfare,' that has resulted in many believing COVID-19 was introduced as a form of biological warfare. Biological weapons are considered a federal crime established under the customary international humanitarian law, and is detailed in most international treaties.

Biological warfare has utilized some of the most well-known infective agents to stage war on others. An example of this was the British army that thought it would be a good idea to use smallpox against the Native Americans. This form of biological warfare was used during the Siege of Fort Pitt in 1763. With the incoming of World War II, there was a ministry of supply in the United Kingdom that wanted to weaponize a large variety of different infective agents. This research was led by Winston Churchill, who had successfully weaponized anthrax, brucellosis, and botulism toxins. The effect of anthrax as a tool of biological warfare was seen most readily at the battle of Gruinard Island in Scotland, with the duration of anthrax infection lasting 56 years.

As technology has advanced, there has been a very strong will to create agents of biological warfare that creates a genetic change in the foe's human body. However, with the use of biotechnology, an endless multitude of different disease causing organisms can be created. A few examples of how biological warfare can alter the role of one's genetics, are as follows:

- A novel virus or bacteria can be equipped with a means to render the effects of a previous vaccine ineffective.
- Biologically crafted warfare agents can alter one's genetics in such a way that resistance to antibiotics and antiviral agents occurs more readily.
- With the use of biotechnology, the virulence of the infective agent is increased, with or without an increase in the degree of transmissibility of the agent. One of the main aims of biological warfare is to ensure

as many people get infected as possible, which is why there is a focus on the degree of transmissibility of the biological agent.

Biological warfare can be a scary aspect of life, especially with how much this pandemic has changed our lives, some permanently. Many share these beliefs on social media, claiming that the COVID-19 virus is an act of biological warfare or a form of government control. However, this specific conspiracy theory has been proven false as there are no specific individuals targeted by COVID-19.

Chapter 6: Rise of Streaming & Gaming Services

COVID-19 has caused a severe strain on the economy; however, one sector that has actually thrived during this period is streaming and gaming services. When stay-at-home orders and lockdowns were announced all over the world, there was a massive wave of people flocking to various streaming services, as well as TV and video game console companies seeing a significant increase in purchases.

We have seen a large spike in gaming activity with many being able to work from home, meaning more time has been spent streaming and playing video games. The average percentage difference between weekdays and weekends was normally 1.5% before COVID-19. However, with the implementation of restrictions, this percentage dropped to 0.56%.

There was even research done on the amount of in-app purchases that occurred. These purchases included microtransactions, especially on mobile games. Individuals yearned for entertainment to keep them busy, which makes sense given that March and April 2020 recorded the highest levels of microtransactions occuring. Not only was the amount of in-app surges increasing, but there was an 84% increase in the amount of mobile applications that were being downloaded. It is these increases that were constant across different countries, especially when compared to the timing of stay-at-home restrictions being implemented. China and Italy, being the first two countries to implement a lockdown, were the first to show surges of up to 50% more traffic than usual. This was the period that app developers needed to take advantage of, especially seeing as more individuals would be relying on technology during this time.

Another reason why there has been a large increase in the amount of time spent on streaming services and video games, is because there is a mental health aspect to it. Many individuals find that video games, or watching their favorite television series, puts them in a world that is of their control. Not only that, by being able to enjoy these adventures with your friends, or even hosting a watch party together, has changed the negative extent that has come with COVID-19.

Regarding the different types of games that were downloaded, there was a spike seen with what is called 'commuter' mobile applications. These applications are those that people typically use to pass the time while commuting to a destination. Not only do these types of games offer shorter play sessions, but they have a level-based system that makes them difficult to put down when playing. Some examples of these games include Candy Crush Saga, Animal Crossing, and your typical arcade games like Pac-man. Just as there was an increase in mobile games, for those seasoned video game veterans, there was an increase in the purchasing and playing of what we call 'Triple A' titles.

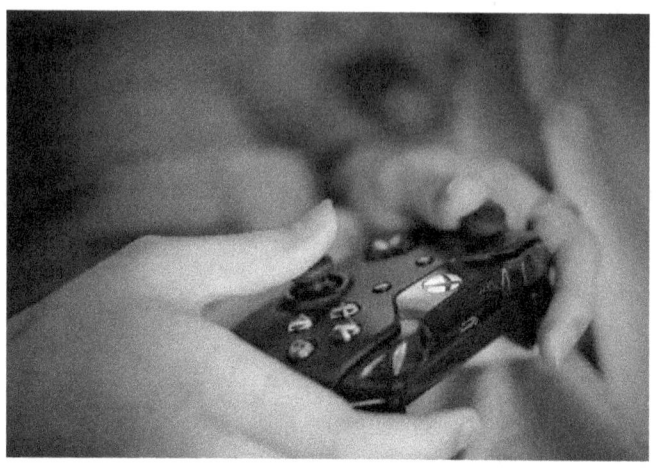

Social networking applications increased by 83%, especially those that offered video call extensions. TikTok became one of the fastest growing social media platforms in history, primarily because it not only offered entertainment, but it allowed others to engage with a wide variety of different communities. Usually social media applications decrease during the summer months, however, seeing as nobody was going on holiday, the traffic that was seen reached world-breaking levels. If only we knew that the COVID-19 pandemic was going to happen, then we would have invested in shares of Zoom and Amazon, seeing as the use of these applications have also shown an insurmountable increase during the pandemic. The primary cause of this is due to the need for platforms that allow one to work remotely and attend meetings. These platforms are used to host virtual birthday parties where lockdown restrictions prevented social gatherings from occurring.

It is no surprise that there has been a surge in online streaming during COVID-19. With the annual study done in the United Kingdom, there was more than 40% of a persons waking hours being spent watching a series, playing video games, or watching videos. The amount of time spent on subscription streaming services doubled during COVID-19, more specifically during April 2020 as that was when most of the countries started to initiate their lockdown regulations. There was also an overall increase in 31% of time spent in front of a screen during waking hours. We have found there was an increase in streaming services such as Netflix, Amazon Prime Video, and Hulu, the average being 71 minutes per day. They also saw an increase of 12 million new subscribers; out of this figure, three million had never used any subscription service before. Adults have also roped in approximately 45 hours a week watching television and online videos (especially YouTube). This led to an increase of 71% in terms of viewing figures when compared to data obtained in 2019.

There has even been an increase in public service broadcasting. In 2020, BBC saw a 59% increase in viewership, the highest increase to have occurred within a six year period. Logically, the main reason for this increase has been due to the public trusting these broadcasting stations for updates regarding not only the status of the COVID-19 pandemic, but also new restrictions that are being imposed. It is expected that as soon as lockdown regulations begin to ease, that there will be a decline in not only the time that the public spends on their screens, but also the amount of individuals that are subscribed to streaming services. In America, the same trend can be seen. MSNBC showed a 12% increase in viewership when comparing 2019 data to 2020, where most of the customers responsible for this increase said they were watching it purely for

COVID-19 updates. Other news broadcasting stations such as CNN and Fox News also showed increases in viewership for the same reasons as MSNBC, increasing at 5% and 14% respectively.

What has now been discovered is that the market size value of video streaming has hit an all time high, with it being worth $50.1 billion. If it were to increase within the steady state, as well as in the predicted linear fashion, come 2027, the revenue forecast for the video streaming industry will amount to $184.2 billion. The types of streaming types that are included within this market are streaming type outlooks, solution outlooks, platform outlooks, service outlooks, revenue model outlooks, and regional outlooks.

The degree at which an established market, such as that of video game services and streaming services, have created levels of income for individuals, is astronomical. An example of this is the TikTok creator fund that pays TikTok creators based on the amount of views their videos get, which is directly impacted by the amount of followers they have. An example of this is TikTok user 'kallmekris' that has taken the market by storm, creating a community that has changed her life. Although we can focus on the detriment that the COVID-19 pandemic, it has shown life-changing opportunities for others. Moving a bit further away from social media, video game streaming services such as Twitch, have shown many individuals braving the online world not only in search of a community, but also as a measure of self-confidence.

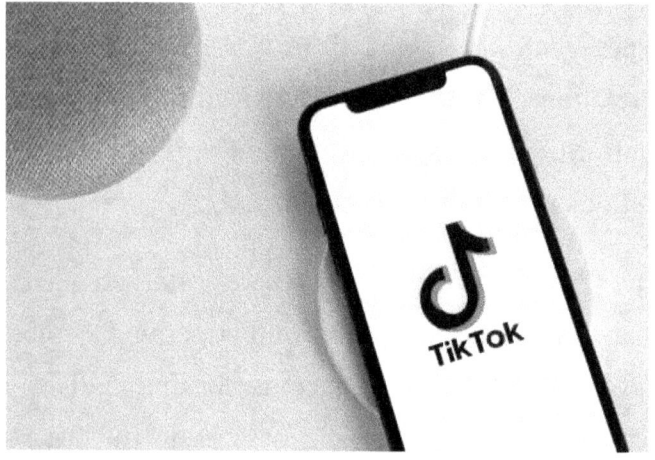

It's easy to overlook the bias against video games and those that stream gameplay online. The stigma is that the content creator is a weird loner who prefers to be separate from others. Now this may be true in some cases, however, many use these platforms to overcome their mental health struggles by making friends online. There are so many people that have acquired a support base online, and gained more friendships than they would in real life (IRL). Not only do they find these online groups of individuals relatable, but many use playing video games as a manner to cope with any levels of inherent stress.

Benefits of Regular Video Game Play

There has been this backlash towards the effects that playing video games has on the cognitive ability of children and adults. It was even during the times of COVID-19 that many families refused to allow any form of video games to be played, despite the need to keep kids busy during lockdown. Studies on the benefits of playing video games have shown the many positive benefits of playing video games. COVID-19 is ultimately creating individuals with stronger cognition skills.

There is typically a direct proportionality present between the degree of coordination that is experienced, along with the amount of time that is spent playing video games. Many assume your mind is blank while staring into a computer screen. However, many of the actions that appear on the screen trigger mental stimulation. It requires the coordination of one's visual, auditory and physical movements. To an extent, this is also why there is such a large feeling of satisfaction when a game is completed after many hours of slow advancement.

Problem-solving skills are heightened, especially in individuals that play puzzle-based video games. Video games, more often than not, involve certain instruction. This requires the player to think critically, informatively, and realistically. Not only does split-second decisions need to be made in specific circumstances, but the ability to think on your feet is also tested. Not only are your problem-solving skills expanded, but you are taught consequences for wrong choices.

An individual's memory will definitely be tested as they traverse a layout designed in a video game. Depending on the game type, a certain quest may require that you need to obtain a specific item that only exists in a specific area, so you need to always remain aware of your surroundings as you progress through the game, as you never know when you might need what you have seen. These memory skills are further able to be used outside the video gaming idea, especially when needing to remember tasks that you are informed of in play.

Attention and concentration are vital skills in life, and there is not really a better way to learn them than in a way you will enjoy and can have fun while doing it. Video games have the immense ability to capture the attention of the player, and in some cases for the entirety of the game. It is the want to complete the game successfully that ensures that an attention to detail, as well as a high level of concentration is always present.

Video games have the ability to be a great source of learning to both adults and children. Many different institutions of education have gamified their learning systems, incorporating a competitive aspect within a video game approach. This approach is ingrained within their teaching methodology, and has been proven to improve academic skills by refining attention to detail. Very specific educational video games allow for the enhancement of both the cognitive and creative skills of an adult or child.

The brain speed of children and adults who play video games is remarkably higher than those who never play. Research has shown that both visual and auditory stimuli are processed a lot faster in those that play video games, than those that do not. It sharpens your skills for occupations that require a fine level of detail and patience. The improvement of social skills is a fantastic part of this past time. With there being a constant degree of communication between those that are playing the same video game online, individuals are able to strengthen bonds with other people their age while being able to make new friends.

Chapter 7:
E-Commerce Boom

At the start of the pandemic because there was still so much uncertainty about the virus, a lot of fear and anxiety surrounded basic tasks, especially when it meant venturing into public, which forced a lot of individuals to opt for online shopping as a way to stay safe. This resulted in an increase in the public's use of online retailers such as Amazon, Ebay, and Shopify to buy everything from workout equipment to groceries. In order to reinforce the need for e-commerce, Deloitte conducted a survey where the results showed that only 61% of adults felt safe venturing outside their homes in order to shop.

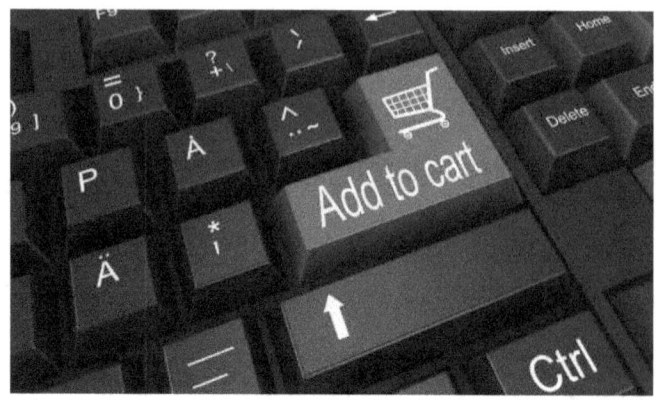

COVID-19 has had an impact on the ability of one to be able to afford specialty items like gifts for birthdays, weddings, or anniversaries. This is primarily due to rampant job cuts, or restructuring companies had to do to stay afloat. A recent study shows that 25% of all consumers experience high levels of stress over not being able to afford the basic necessities. On top of this, 30% of consumers also said that they are going to be spending less this holiday season.

Buy Now, Pay Later

This is where layby businesses have stepped in, ensuring consumers have access to products they need by allowing them to pay later. With the 'buy now, pay later' business model being around for quite some time, the COVID-19 has strengthened its use, especially as those struggling financially required access to resources which they simply could not afford given the current circumstances. The United Kingdom has one of the most integrated 'buy now, pay later' systems in the world, where they cater for those that have both poor and excellent credit scores. There are even options that do not require any form of deposit when making a purchase. A few examples of these offered services are as follows:

- Hughes: This online market is specifically catered for those that are looking for appliances such as washing machines, refrigerators, and even gaming consoles. The reason that they are so popular is because a credit check and initial deposit is not required. Being one of the first businesses to offer an unlimited duration to make payment, they are focused on the practicality of each individual's earning potential and the expenses that they have, allowing as many payments as needed until the entire balance of the item has been cleared.

- Tymit: This online purchasing platform has completely reinvented the definition of 'credit.' Tymit offers fixed payment rates and allows the buyer to choose their installment plan, with there being no added costs should the item be repaid over a period less than three months. Not only are there no early repayment charges, but Tymit further groups your purchases together so you can monitor your spending and protect your credit score.

- Flava: A grocery service that uses its online platform to ensure that you are able to remain healthy whilst shopping at a discounted price. With this platform allowing one to buy bulk at discounted rates, they are a fan favorite in the United Kingdom, readily used by students and in preparation for conferences. With there being a benefit card available, those that use Flava Are able to save up to 30% on all their purchases.

Luckily for some e-commerce institutes like Amazon, negative effects of COVID-19 remained non-existent. With Amazon somehow growing even bigger and securing its sport as the number one e-commerce site on the planet. Their sales nearly doubled by May of 2020. When we look at the comparative growth during this period, Amazon is the third biggest users of digital ads, which provides a very strong revenue stream. With a company maximizing their earning potential, you would expect them to give back to communities in need, especially during this time, and they have. Amazon invested a total of $4 million into COVID-19 prevention programs, and this money went towards purchasing PPE for healthcare workers, and providing cleaning supplies for essential businesses required to stay open during such a dangerous time when death tolls were rising each day.

With the ability of Amazon to effectively monopolize the online market, they are able to appease consumer culture. Give the masses discounts, quick delivery options, and you have a winning business model. This is where the 'Prime' subscription comes in with its many perks. Not only does Amazon Prime offer free two-day delivery, they even offer same day grocery delivery, prescription delivery, and an option to save up to 5% on all purchases. Amazon is able to tap into the multi-domain lifestyle while making lives easier, and keeping people safe during the COVID-19 pandemic.

There have been so many other businesses that capitalized on the COVID-19 pandemic to grow their businesses and provide better services for their users. An example of this is Zoom. This video conferencing app was able to successfully make businesses, schools, and social gatherings happen with one click. In June 2020, Zoom's sales had increased by 169% three consecutive times starting in March, when the entire world needed to convert to working remotely. This further became a necessity as many companies did not allow more than a certain amount of individuals to be physically present at work. From a monetary perspective, by the end of April 2020, Zoom had made $328.2 million, being able to offer more advanced technology to ensure their quality of services remained top tier.

Why Switch to an Online Market?

So, why is everyone moving to e-commerce? What makes the online space that much different than running a brick and mortar business?

When wanting to enter into the e-commerce space, you will figure out that the startup costs associated with beginning your e-commerce venture are rather low. Remember, everything that is done online just needs a stable internet connection. There is no need to dish out large sums of money for rent, electricity and other amenities, when all you have, being your computer, wireless internet, and comfort of your own home, is really all you need. However, if you are thinking of starting your own online store, or even starting your dream of owning your own blog, a website or shopping platform will come with its own set of costs. The list of total expenditure for building a website, will never remain at a constant rate. The price is based on a multitude of different factors which include: how integrated you want your website to be, whether third party systems need to be linked, whether you are creating the content for the website yourself or if you are employing someone else to do it. A basic list of costs involved are as follows:

- Website domain: $12-$60 (depending on where the domain is purchased from, as well as whether it is a dot com, dot org, or country-code website).
- Website hosting: $35-$600 (depending on the type of website, whether automated backups of data are needed, as well as how many monthly visitors you have).
- Secure Sockets Layer (SSL) Certificate: $0-$200.

- Website template or theme: $0-$200 (depending on whether someone is employed to construct the template or theme).
- E-commerce functionality (applicable for online stores only): $20-$24,000.
- Website content: $0-$5000.
- Applications and integrations: $0-$100.
- Search Engine Optimization (SEO) and marketing: $0-$90

Building a website can cost as little as $6 per month when one uses a pre-designed website designer, moving towards up to $10,000 for a web designer to build a site for you. On average, for a rather basic website where minimal online shopping is occurring, the cost is a couple hundred dollars. A maintenance cost of approximately fifty dollars is required to ensure that the website is running smoothly. Many individuals, especially those that want to write blogs, test their skills using free versions of Wordpress and Wix before committing to creating their own website, as it can become rather costly very fast.

There are no set hours of operation with an online business. There is always an opportunity for you to make a sale. Within this space of time, an online store allows you to effectively attract your target market by appealing to what they value - time. Many individuals do not have time to do in-person shopping, so rely on e-commerce for purchases. However, how do online businesses actually generate an income? Many would think that income generated would be purely from sales, however, that is not the case. Here are a few examples of how online businesses generate an income:

- Selling services or physical products: There are many individuals that have taken advantage of the COVID-19 situation, especially that of personal trainers, in providing online coaching for those that have not been able to attend the gym due to lockdown restrictions. Freelancers, lawyers and business consultants further found that

COVID-19 had caused a spike in their customer base. With providing physical products, those that are typically placed on the online platforms are anything that can be created, modified, or purchased for re-selling.

- Information products: These products include ebooks, online video courses, templates, guides, as well as worksheets.
- Donations: Charitable organizations that have an online platform, typically offer the option of being able to donate with their purchase. If one focuses purely on donations and not the providing of a service or physical product, businesses like Patreon allow the public to offer donations to content creators based on the type and frequency of content that they produce. Chapo Trap House and Amanda Palmer are top Patreon creators that earn $95,000 and $55,000 respectively, per month.
- Subscribed communities: The delivery of themed snackboxes has taken the world by

storm. Companies like NatureBox provide this service, focusing on the regular delivery of healthy and nutritious snacks based on a subscription service. One of the most common forms of 'crates' is that of Japan Crate and Bokksu, which provides local delicacies, as well as Anime merchandise to Japanese enthusiasts worldwide. The prices of these subscription boxes typically range from between $14.99 to $34.99 based on the frequency of delivery as well as the types of items that have been requested to be included in the box.

E-commerce does not confine you to selling locally in a physical location. It promotes an international platform to showcase your items. COVID-19 has really allowed the interconnectedness of so many different small business owners, establishing a community that supports each other's growth. All that will need to be factored here is shipping costs associated with a customer's purchase. However, if you are able to tackle a well-known and reputable shipping company that is affordable, there will be no problem in keeping your customer base strong. When one sells internationally, the potential for you to build your own brand increases dramatically. This not only allows you to broaden your marketplace, but it further allows you to visualize your profits rising faster than when compared to a local business who can only cater to a specific group.

As one starts growing their online business, it becomes seemingly impossible to do all of the work on your own. However, one does not need to stress about this as there is direct access to affordable employees. What is a key take away within this domain is that you have a greater pool of expertise as you have the ability to hire from anywhere in the world. You are also able to positively contribute to the livelihoods of many individuals, especially those where the cost of living is lower compared to your own.

As established above, this is the future of commerce especially as we make more time available to work, spend time with family, and pick up new hobbies.

Not only are there critical thought processes behind the applicability in this context, but there are definitive numbers that show the adoption of e-commerce strategies. With the use of statistics, it is predicted that the amount of sales within the global market will reach $4.9 trillion by 2021. When compared to sales since 2014, there are no signs of regression, with a constant and linear pattern. As the trend strengthens, the degree of e-commerce that will occupy the total sales within the global retail market will reach 17.5% by 2021.

COVID-19 has definitely paved the way for growth in e-commerce. However, a tier of e-commerce that is currently growing at an exponential rate, due to the impact of the pandemic is social media shopping. Those that are social sellers, have such a large chance of integrating their sales with Facebook ads, as well as sponsored posts on Instagram. With the amount of individuals that have used their lockdown practices as a means to involve themselves in the trenches of social media, the chances of seeing these adverts may increase dramatically. Seeing as many individuals highly discount the effects and power of social media, some do not do research regarding the benefits thereof. With so many of these social shopping e-commerce enterprises appearing, a similar tact that has been rolled out is the 'purchase' button that allows one to shop directly on the application whilst scrolling through social media. For instance, Instagram introduced 'shoppable posts' which show you how much the items on a picture are simply by tapping it. What they will typically see is an image of the product, a very brief description of the product, the price, as well as a link that will take them to the website where the product can be purchased.

E-commerce trends therefore cut both the time, as well as that of the effort needed when shoppers want to use social media as a purchasing platform. COVID-19 has brought in a new era of social selling, and everyone is adapting to this change by spending as little time as possible ordering their goods while maximizing the saved time by taking care of other more pressing tasks. COVID-19, using this adaptability to change, has resulted in a global shift of the center of e-commerce from that of the western hemisphere, towards a more widespread European and Eastern localization. This shift means that businesses need to start to tailor the goods and services they offer towards a more international standpoint. Not only does this impart a sense of global accessibility and convenience to the customer, but a global business model will further ensure that you have access to external goods and services that your country of residence does not necessarily have.

If you are well aware that your market is global, but have no idea how this market can be reached, COVID-19 has resulted in the presence of a lot of businesses that specialize in integrating products into countries and the global markets where they were not previously present. An example is Mondelez International, which partners with a business called ChannelSight. This ensured that the goods (Oreos and Cadbury) reached a total of 25 new markets that spanned across more than 130 retailer websites.

COVID-19's benefits within the e-commerce sector have proven that seemingly catastrophic situations, including a pandemic, have the potential to bear fruit that can positively change the lives of others. By doing a quick search, you are able to see the growth of this industry, as well as recognize the need of these facilities in the modern day. The need for technological markets that are expressed using online platforms, has shown through during this time of the COVID-19 pandemic. So, if you have been looking for a new enterprise to start making money, why not try online?

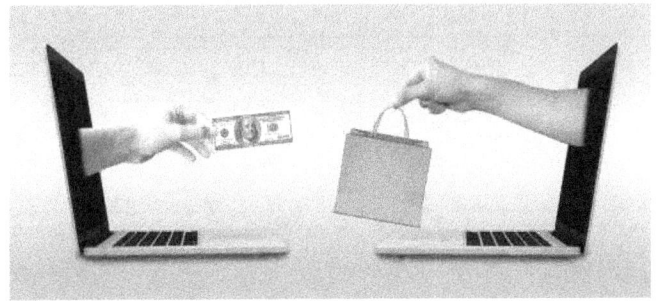

Chapter 8: Electronic Payment Systems

As e-commerce escalated during the COVID-19 pandemic, what was also found was that the electronic payment systems that had started to be integrated within these platforms peaked rather quickly. The opportunities for electronic payment systems to flourish within the context of new e-commerce businesses, is really what has driven the benefit of COVID-19 to the general public. American Express is seen as being a pretty big electronic payment service provider, Furthermore, what they have seen, especially in the last few months of the pandemic, is that there has been more than a 90% increase in the amount of payments that are being made. Naturally, this is due to the exponential increase in the amount of online shopping that has occurred.

The expectation is that these numbers are most likely going to continue rising, especially as the development of new digital categories start to saturate the e-commerce market. With COVID-19 having exposed the gaps within the e-commerce system, businesses are taking this as a major advantage to get stuck into the market. With many of the fintech evangelists establishing a sense of credited demonetization, the presence of COVID-19 has definitely changed their approach towards the e-commerce industry. What the COVID-19 pandemic really has done is to expedite the evolution and adoption of technologically centered modes of online payment that provide a requirement for the general public.

However, there is a definitive paradigm shift in the manner that a customer behaves. This is based on the types of payments that they use for services and subscriptions that they are assigned to. What was found included that online shopping was not just used for purchasing via stores such as Amazon and Etsy, and that the payment of one's utility bills, health and fitness subscriptions, as well as insurance premiums have all been switched to transacting online. In some countries there is even an option to pay your parking tickets using a country-based mobile application. There used to be this fear that those in older generations would struggle in adopting these new electronic payment services. However, the COVID-19 pandemic has inadvertently forced individuals to understand how these transactions are to work. What COVID-19 has taught us is that the development within the context of digital financial services are mandatory and necessary to maintain each individual's livelihood.

The COVID-19 pandemic has further resulted in the surfacing of some business potholes, especially within the context of American Express. This electronic payment service has been trying to rid the image that it is only meant for the elite. The reason for this is that they started to lose a bit of customer traction within the COVID-19 pandemic, especially from middle class workers that believed they were not 'American Express material.' The adaptive nature of American Express will definitely need to shine through, especially with the development of other fintech companies that are gearing and focussing their efforts towards providing virtual card services.

With COVID-19 having accelerated at the degree in which digital payment services are being adopted, many fintech businesses that focus on electronic payments are found targeting the same users. Not only does this narrow the playing field, but if the correct marketing approach is not followed, it could lead to early bankruptcy. With this being said, COVID-19 has caused businesses to do some serious introspection regarding their operational costs and an analysis as to barriers that are hindering their growth.

Moving a bit further away from the seemingly elite, Visa and Mastercard have gained much traction within the context of COVID-19. With many banks utilizing Visa and Mastercard services for online purchasing, it is not to be expected that there is such an increase in not only their dividends, but also their growth patterns during the pandemic.

However, although many banks are affiliated with either Visa or Mastercard because of their similarities they are typically grouped together within the same category of electronic payments. Many individuals have this idea that they are one and the same, however, there are indeed small differences that COVID-19 has effectively highlighted.

With the education market tapping into the disadvantages of credit cards and emphasizing them, there has been a direct preference for debit cards over and above credit cards. When comparing the services that Visa and Mastercard have to offer, there is a heightened favor of debit-based services offered by Visa. Based on this fact, there has been a heightened volume of debit transactions, constituting a further 52% of total card-based transactions. This specific value of Visa was compared to the 44% of total card-based transactions from Mastercard. When establishing reasons as to why Visa has seen such a large increase in the amount of swipes, is primarily because COVID-19 has imposed a replacement cash with card, which is made easily available by the more debit-centered Visa electronic payment service.

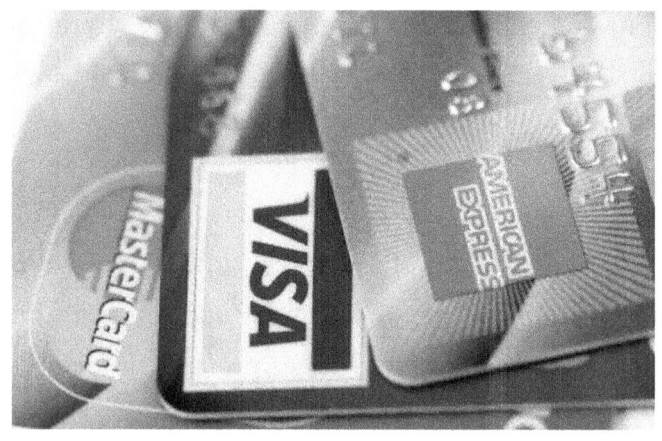

COVID-19 has caused individuals to tend closer towards switching purely towards completing transactions using cards instead of cash. The reason for this is because COVID-19 has got many individuals very hesitant regarding touching any form of cash, with there being a fear that COVID-19 could be transmitted in this way. When we compare the total rise in debit cards being used, it is evidently seen that both Visa and Mastercard have had reputable growth of up to 20% their normal amounts. However, the reason that we have Visa gaining a lot more momentum than Mastercard, is based on the degree of debit that facilitates a larger area of spend within a business. As time progresses, there is a suspicion that as the amount of debit transactions increase, the amount of credit transactions will decrease.

However, analysts are foreshadowing that there will only be an inverse occurring many years after COVID-19 as it does not favor the needs of the current climate that the world finds itself in. What was further established was that the COVID-19 pandemic has resulted in the inclusion of another dynamic. This dynamic is the definitive shift towards debit only transactions, especially seeing as the pandemic has caused the direct movement from cash to cards. This change establishes a strengthened debit value that the individual has direct access to without any external fees.

Many local electronic payment services have partnered with Visa and Mastercard in order to allow small business owners a greater earning potential during the pandemic. An example of this is Yoco, a card machine that connects via bluetooth to any smartphone, where the amount is typed on the phone and registered on the bluetooth device. With the card machine being able to fit in the palm of your hand, it provides both card-based and tap technology. Thus, it is important to realize that there has been a severe impact on third world countries, and the small informal businesses that are operating. With this in mind, Yoco believed it was a good idea to add towards the COVID-19 cause by implementing measures with their products to prevent the spread. For third world countries, there has been a greater need for quick transitions, resulting in entrepreneurs needing to adapt immediately to remain competitive in the bustling market.

With Yoco playing a pivotal role in allowing others to be able to contribute positively to the economy in South Africa, they instilled a multiple step process that can be adopted to keep accounts balanced throughout the lockdown period, providing points that need to be thought of in order to ensure whether the operation of your business is viable in a post-COVID-19 context.

Managing your expenses is one of the first aspects that need to be considered, especially if COVID-19 has placed you in a predicament where your country is under a strict lockdown and you are unable to open your business. There needs to be some deep introspection where an analysis needs to take place that ranks your expenses based on their importance in keeping things operational. Many businesses draw up this list through bank statements and receipts to remove all unnecessary expenditures. A useful way that this is done (which may require some research on your part) is to divide all of the expenses that you have into either fixed, periodical, or variable. Not only will this method allow you to better understand your expenses, but it will further enable you to manage your budget effectively.

You want to ensure that a business forecast is made based on the current financial status of the company. This is why it is recommended that a foreshadow of three months is performed based on the ever-changing environment that the COVID-19 pandemic has placed us in. A forecasted budget will allow for expense adjustments to be made, relative to the amount of shortfalls that present itself.

During the pandemic any revenue brought in means there is a lesser chance of shortfalls that can lead to permanent closure. It doesn't hurt to have a revenue strategy plan in place in order to ensure that the safety requirements for the public are adhered to. The more you focus on your businesses' COVID-19 adapted target market with research, you will ensure the prices charged for your goods and services will be enough to keep your business afloat throughout the ups and downs of the pandemic. If you can no longer operate your business during lockdown, use this time to think of ways that revenue can be enhanced by exploring new income sources.

Fine Tune Your Business Model

In order to ensure that your business is being run effectively, use this extra time to analyze and fine-tune your business model, as this is the only way you will be able to develop an improved product cost to profit ratio which allows enough runway for your business to function despite COVID-19.

A few questions that you can ask yourself include:

- What does the length of my financial runway look like?
- Is there a possibility that I can establish enough sales to get through lockdown without any extra means of funding?
- Are there any cuts I can make to the business to ensure it remains cost-effective?
- What other sources of income can I look into to ensure your business remains funded during the time of COVID-19?
- Is there potential to seek formal funding for my business such as a small business loan?

What COVID-19 has taught us, and this applies to the electronic payment services domain as well, is that there is always hope for being able to get out of tough situations. All you need to do is seek solutions to problems by tackling the already existing business issues, and transforming them into strategic business gains that places you further ahead than your competitors.

This is exactly what happened with PayPal, as they found themselves decreasing their holding potential for their clients, and if servers would be able to manage the influx of new customers that COVID-19 brought with it. PayPal has actually had an increased financial return this year. Data from September shows more than 10 million new accounts have been created, with 9.3 million more accounts than 2019 in the same time period. When COVID-19 caused the implementation of the stringent lockdown protocols across the world in April, 7.4 million new accounts were created. This latter value has been the greatest growth that PayPal has seen since inception. Based on further data, there were 451 studies performed which reinforced the increase in the PayPal app being downloaded. With there not being a premium account option, PayPal's resources are made available to everyone from businesses paying employees, private contractors able to send invoices, to friends sending money for a small fee. Even with COVID-19, this company has managed to hold the top digital money transfer spot.

Electronic payment services have increased throughout COVID-19, while increasing the amount of business opportunities for entrepreneurs. Electronic payment services have changed how we approach buying online. What this provides is more time we would not have had if we purchased items and services in-person. The benefits that these online payment services have on accessibility outweighs any of the grievances others may have.

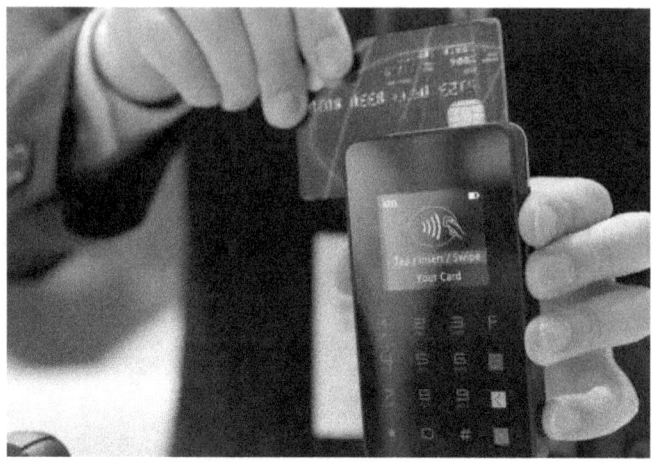

Chapter 9:
The Telecommunication Industry

The telecommunication industry has increased dramatically during COVID-19 as everyone is looking for ways to stay connected while being safe at home. In order for us to understand the extent at which the telecommunication industry has been impacted by COVID-19, we should look at what it entails. It integrates both telephone companies and your internet service providers, two factors that have become a major part of our lives during this pandemic.

Due to the increase in lockdown restrictions imposed within each country and as borders closed across the world, a demand for social and work connections has risen. There is now a specific focus on increasing a network's ability to hold a strong video connection to replace person to person contact. And within the medical sphere, this data has been used to track the progression and extent of the COVID-19 spread. Reliability of each network has been the focus for progression, even beyond the pandemic. However, with the massive influx of app servers as COVID-19 shut everything down, the telecommunications industry faced its first string of issues. These were handled by lowering the pixel quality of video, the sound quality of voice calls, as well as the rebuffering of streams decreased.

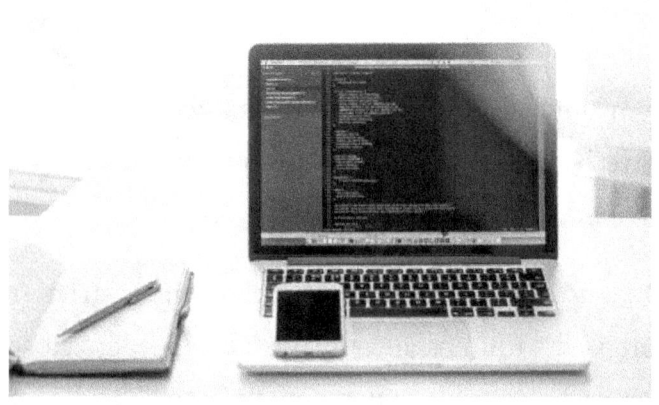

With so many recurring changes and updates within this domain, there were definitely a few changes that the customer would experience. Telecommunication industries have increased their capacity, which in many instances resulted in an increase in usage speeds by the customer. In April 2020, Korea showed an increased bandwidth usage of 13%, leading to a total of 60% of their deployed internet capacity being utilized at any given moment. NTT Communications in Japan documented a 65% surge in their bandwidth usage during May 2020, with internet speeds of users decreasing dramatically. In Italy, a COVID-19 stricken area, Telecom Italia showed an increase in data usage of more than 63% between April 2020 and June 2020. As a turn around, many data and internet service providers opened up for unlimited minutes, reassured there would be no direct cuts of data supplies. The first company to do this was AT&T as they had noticed a 42% increase of Wi-Fi usage, resulting in their core network traffic accounting for 23% of the total data usage in America in May of this year.

Other lesser known businesses within the umbrella of the telecommunication industry wanted to provide users an opportunity to use their tools free of charge. An example was Creative Cloud that was supplied by Adobe to be free for both students and teachers in order to allow effective distanced learning to take place. Adobe offered free versions of Adobe Portfolio, Adobe Lightroom, and Adobe Spark to all students during COVID-19.

The use of tracked data with track and trace programs such as England's NHS Covid-19 app by the government to follow and help contain the spread of COVID-19 as a protective protocol, needed to be 100% accurate. With the mass COVID-19 screening procedures, the need for high quality and efficient telecom businesses could not be overlooked. Apple is also in the works with Google to release an in-home screening process for evaluating potential infections. All with the goal to alleviate already overcrowded hospitals With the use of GPS enabled tracking to monitor the movements of those that have been infected with COVID-19, and ensure they are remaining isolated, it leads many to the question the fairness of these practices and if this accumulated data will remain private and secure within the telecomm services.

One way to combat these fears and stay ahead of any privacy leaks, we have seen the integration of 5G network speeds within the time period of COVID-19, and as you would guess the adoption has not been as smooth as with fiber optic internet connections.

The Future of 5G

The worldwide 5G telecommunications market is set to encounter a negative effect in 2020, primarily due to the introduction of the COVID-19 pandemic. When we take a further look at the expanding ventures for building frameworks that focus specifically on 5G innovation, it is anticipated to hamper the telecommunications market until the time-frame of COVID-19 being abolished is reached. One of the main roots of inaccessibility stems from the 5G gadgets not being made as available as necessary in order for electronics to run and operate effectively. What this further does is completely cut off the abilities of others with less advanced technology to communicate with others. As the development of 5G comes into play, it will result in upgrades and modifications needing to be made in order to cater for the new service. This will require the abolishment of less effective services, such as 3G as it is not only too expensive, but the ratio of individuals using that service does not cover the costs involved with keeping that service active.

Studies about the 5G infrastructure market have utilized statistics to predict a set revenue by 2027, consisting of $41 million, with a steady growth rate of 64.6% during a 10 year period. These numbers were not just calculated using average data, but focused on integrating the operational frequency of 5G infrastructure, with that of the region in order to establish a set segmental analysis of where regional 5G infrastructure fits in the global market. With this being said, there is an expected increase in mobile data traffic that will drive the transition into the 5G framework of data supply. Where careful consideration needs to be acknowledged, is based on the degree at which the 5G technology may hamper the telecommunication industry's market if instituted within the thicket of COVID-19.

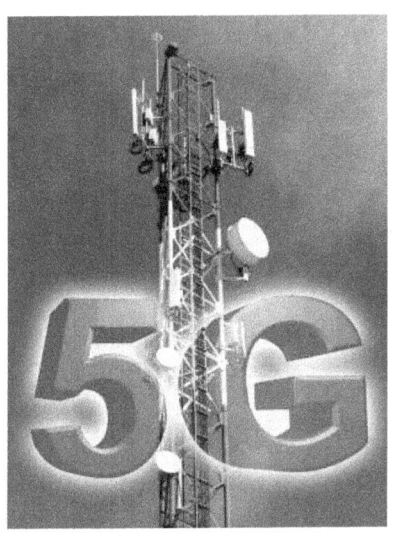

This is mainly due to the speculation that still exists within the public domain, with 5G said to be a part of the controlling nature of COVID-19 as a biological warfare tactic, which is honestly absurd.

The telecommunication industry has had quite a surge in online grocery shopping amidst the pandemic. The main reason for this was that people were just too scared and anxious to go and perform in-person shopping. What this unfortunately led to, was the stockpile mentality that was seen worldwide. A study done in China showed that fresh food e-commerce channels had resulted in a more prominent incidence of panic stockpiling. The reason for this increased likelihood was due to the supply shortages that were suspected, especially seeing as the government had begun to take over tenders and the logistic management that underpinned the importing of essential goods. Furthermore, when the researchers decided to look at 'community group buying,' which is another class of e-commerce and the telecommunication industry, the needs were fulfilled easier. Psychologists believe that the reason for this is on the premise that one knows that everyone is getting the same amount of an item, ameliorating any thoughts of there being a perception of panic buying within the community.

The telecommunication industry, in collaboration with COVID-19, has resulted in the search for more diverse channels to obtain goods. Not only was it important that the most cost effective options were offered, but that there was an open channel to provide a constant flow of goods and services. This sparked online channels to develop a reputable means to supply goods and services during extreme situations, with which the response from the government would not have been as instantaneous as using an online trading platform. This prompted companies around the world to keep the private sector stable by including both the new and increased online grocery and sales marketplaces, as well as the traditional offline channels that had already established a profitable reputation before the impact of COVID-19.

The amount of telecommunication industry request spikes resulted in the prompting of momentary income upticks, especially from those that use data as an integral part of providing their business services, as well as the internet service providers. The amount of growth experienced within the COVID-19 time period continues today, offering some relief within the industry. It wass expected that COVID-19 would result in the shutting down of businesses, but whenever you take a step backwards and acknowledge the silver-lining within the telecommunication industry, the COVID-19 pandemic has revealed business markets and opportunities that were never noticeable before seeing as most of the current world's population has not lived through a pandemic.

What COVID-19 has prompted is the necessity for an evolution of business practice advancements that utilize an adaptable approach that provides its users what they need. A huge advantage when thinking of connective services, whether it be voice or video, is the unpredictability and constant fine-tuning required to keep up with the worldwide trends that influence the economy as we know it. With the degrees of different lockdown in each country, the development of salesmen and wholesalers saw an evident spike. However, what we actually saw, due to COVID-19, was a halt place on the worldwide economy. Not only did this harbor normal and routine transactions, butit placed a barrier between a business' ability to bring in new clients. This was due to the unclear nature of where the economy and telecommunication industry will be five years from now.

What COVID-19 has done is make it extremely difficult for individuals to save money, based on the irregular income streams that have continued. This is why many have strived to create a sense of harmony between satisfying their basic needs, while saving money on the off chance there is an extended financial slump that has been caused by the pandemic. Through there being a financial slump, there has been a mass exposure of one's vulnerabilities, especially within the financial domain of the telecommunications industry. What has further transpired is how businesses have begun to rely heavily on individuals to maintain their support, even during financially strained times. This has placed pressure on the customers that are unable to afford internet, unlimited data, and subscription services. In terms of 5G, there are many individuals that just cannot afford the switch, which ultimately results in the possibility of many being left behind.

Many businesses in television have begun to focus solely on broadcasting news of financial strain, which was to be expected with such a sweeping loss for so many. The pandemic has resulted in season cancellations for almost every sport across the world, and many of these businesses relying on advertisements to generate revenue to stay afloat. Naturally, many of these types of businesses consisted of long-term investments that they could tap into as a resource in order to address any financial shortfalls that may have started to present itself.

COVID-19 has played a pivotal role in introducing the fourth industrial revolution by referring to all the new technology and treatment modalities being researched, using equipment that many did not even know existed. By utilizing this pandemic as a method of sensitizing businesses to the concept of the fourth industrial revolution, there have been doors opened for businesses to identify new solutions for existing problems within their given field. It has been through this time of COVID-19 that computerized interchange stations have demonstrated the importance of heaping a central human culture within many businesses and industries. Not only did this result in many to feel more grounded, but it also contributed to an increase in their productivity levels.

The telecommunications industry, with its different domains, has both taken the hardest of hits, but also proved the greatest of increases. The ability for people to work from home during the COVID-19 pandemic may have been the biggest benefit. Research shows that individuals that move into the telecommunication industry are likely introverts who prefer to manage their own time, and work better in their home space. This demonstrates the degree at which introverts increase their own productivity in areas that they find themselves comfortable. With them now focusing on work within the comfort of their homes, with access to food and drinks they enjoy, they have acclimatized readily towards the changes the COVID-19 pandemic has brought.

The view from the public now more than ever is the importance of staying connected and consider it a necessity. Let us take a step back and think about what would have happened if we experienced the COVID-19 pandemic in the 1800s. There was no form of medical technology, as well as there being no exact form of direct communication without physically arriving at someone else's house. Thus, if we look retrospectively at what could have happened, we need to acknowledge that the growth and beginning of modern industry has not only allowed us to work remotely, but it has also reinforced the ingrained nature of how we view technology in our lives. If we were to remove all forms of technology from our daily routine, even if it was just for one day, we would begin to realize how easy our lives actually are.

It is of no surprise that our wired society continues to grow in such a way. What we do not know is the extent at which this growth will directly influence our lives. In this day and age, most people's homes, even diverse in age, strictly rely on the flow of information to continue running smoothing. When you see a blip or shortage in this instant access, it indefinitely halts the day. This is why the telecom industry continues to grow. What we see is that there is a direct interplay between the need for newer technology, as well as the ability of the large telecommunication industries to provide us with what we want. With technology, there is never an 'enough' there is always an adaptation that can be implemented that modifies the approach that we take towards integrating technology into our lives.

What if we did not have the internet, mobile data, video game calling services, or social media? Where would we be? This is why technological innovations are so important, even more so when speaking on the future of society and our continual dealings with COVID-19. It allows us to feel connected, speaking to friends and family in another town, or on the other side of the world. It has changed the way that we live, and we should take more time to appreciate the advances that these advantages do for us, ensuring we always have what we need, whether it be groceries, a christmas present, or a FaceTime chat with grandma. This brings us to our next point, the people behind the screens.

Chapter 10:
What About Us?

We cannot forget that, we, the people that have witnessed the full effect of COVID-19. Our mental health has suffered, our savings have run dry, and many have lost loved ones due to COVID-19. This is not something we are equipped to handle on our own, this situation is distressing and luckily more of this supportive message is being spread and acknowledged by the masses: we need your help. There will always be a sense of dread and tension as this dangerous time drags on. General well-being practices like self-isolation can cause individuals to feel just that, alone and hopeless, increasing the potential for anxiety, depression, and apprehension about what the future holds for us; if we will ever get back on track. By following proper sanitation practices, maintaining distance, and checking in with each other as often as we can, is how we will 'flatten the curve,' as well as maintain our mental health.

Stress is one of the key feelings that COVID-19 has heightened, allowing many to realize the pressure they experience, even if they believe they are immune to stress or have never felt the effects as deeply as others. The impacts of stress very, and can include anything from:

- An increase in worry over the well-being of yourself, your friends, colleagues, extended family, and your financial status.
- The future of the job market and what that looks like as COVID-19 progresses.
- Changes in sleep patterns and eating habits.
- Having trouble with thinking clearly and focusing on one specific task.
- Development of chronic medical conditions, or flare-ups of those already present.
- Strained psychological conditions associated with mental health.
- An increase in the use of tobacco, liquor, or other illicit substances.

How you react to pressure during this time relies on a multitude of factors like your maturity level, mental state, degree of social interaction you have with your partner (if married) and family, as well as your financial means.

Lockdowns can elicit a state of emergency within your mind. Not only does this keep your body in a level of high-alert, but it also has the potential to decrease your immune system and make you more prevalent to other infections. That's why it's important to pay attention to what you are eating on a daily basis and to make smart choices. Be sure to include more than the usual amount of vegetables and consider a supplement regimen to make up for any loss of vitamins and minerals. Consult with a doctor on this beforehand to make sure your body gets what it needs.

Interacting with your friends and family can relieve pressure or feelings of loss you may experience. However, seeing as COVID-19 has the potential to infect anyone, you may find the act of helping others adapt as a meaningful, almost therapeutic act. Some might not have access to food, or don't want to risk regular trips to the grocery store or market. If you are healthy, and feel confident in your ability to go out in public and avoid infection, offer to grocery shop for these individuals and even pitch in more sanitizing products for their peace of mind when retrieving these items. Giving to others in need, provides a sense of fulfillment and pride in your abilities to make a difference, resulting in a serotonin boost we could all use. Also voice or video calls to neighbors and grandparents play an immensely supportive role in making these people feel special and important, when otherwise they have felt forgotten.

Here are some other ways that you can alleviate pressures that the COVID-19 pandemic may be ushering onto you:

- Establish what basic necessities you require should you feel the need to isolate or are required to self-quarantine for two weeks. This extends beyond food and toiletries, anything from spa treatments to puzzles, e-readers, or video games. Find things to keep your mind busy and your soul satiated.

- Boost mental wellness. Adopt breathing techniques and meditation practices to help clear your mind if daily life begins to weigh on your conscious. You can use apps such as Breathe and Insight Timer to help you finely tune these activities.

- Retain or maintain good hygiene and wellness. Make sure to go to bed at a reasonable hour, and make it a habit (weekends too!). If you are working from home, wake up in the morning and make your bed, get dressed, and spend time in an area other than your bedroom laying down to boost productivity. Avoid defaulting to scrolling on your phone during downtime or if you get bored. We will go into more detail below with the 'four pillars.'

- Ensure that the information that you are viewing on social media and on the news comes from a trusted source, and always do your research. There are a lot of fake news sites out there looking to turn a profit and don't but the reader first. As soon as you start feeding yourself the negative perspectives that surround COVID-19, you can unknowingly cause a spike in your stress levels and anxiety.

- Know where and how to get treatment if you become sick. Look online for in-person consultations available in your immediate area if you prefer to avoid hospitals, or if your insurance covers telehealth services. Remember to always consult a healthcare professional before you start any self-treatment for an infection.

Psychological well-being is a significant part of a person's functioning. When we are emotionally unwell we tend to seek isolation more, as well as tend to overthink even the most simple of tasks. This becomes a problem, especially in the middle of a pandemic. Not only does a positive sense of psychological well-being ensure that we are less stressed, but it further influences how we feel, think and act.

Individuals with conditions that are directly related to poor mental health or substance abuse, may feel rather helpless in the face of a pandemic and these effects may be exacerbated by the fact. This is due to the negative sense of hopelessness that underlines a tendency to act out. Some examples of chronic conditions that affect one's mental health include: anxiety, depression, bipolarism, schizophrenia, and feeling constantly delirious.

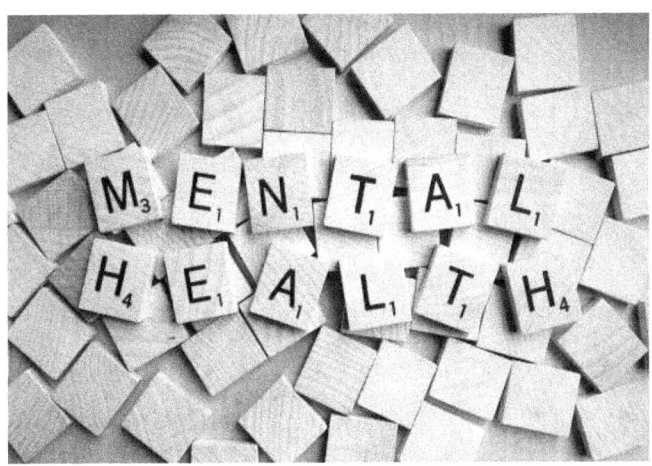

In order for you to effectively tap into your inner positivity, as well as avoid the repercussions of a negative outlook it's important to take time to stay present, stay relaxed, and give yourself time to recuperate when necessary. There are a few methods that focus on providing you a healthier approach to your emotions. Following these will allow you to strengthen your response to the pandemic, cementing a positive focus on what's important, you.

The Four Pillars

You can develop unshakable willpower towards COVID-19 by putting effort into maintaining the 'four pillars.' These pillars are restful sleep, regulated nutrition, socializing, and regular physical fitness. For a holistic sense of well-being to be achieved, these four pillars resemble the legs of a table and need to remain in good condition for the body to properly operate. In the event that one breaks, our emotions can react and our mental health is more likely to suffer. Tapping into the ideals of these four legs will help us answer commonly asked questions. With this we can reveal where there are potential gaps in our mental health that need immediate attention.

Restful Sleep

When we deal with the concept of sleep it is more than just getting six or eight hours. What you want to do, is measure the amount of quality sleep that is obtained. To better measure your sleep patterns and improve, ask yourself:

- What time do you normally fall asleep? How long after you get into bed does it take you to fall asleep? Do you believe you are maintaining a healthy sleep schedule?
- While asleep, how often do you wake up during the night?
- What can you do to improve these patterns?
- Do you take naps during the day? How long do they typically last? Naps that exceed 20 minutes typically interrupt your sleep patterns by telling your body it's time to

sleep and will attempt to put you in a REM cycle. This will leave you feeling groggy and tired for the rest of the day.

- How many hours do you spend on your phone while laying in bed before you fall asleep or wake up in the morning?

Regulated Nutrition

The nutritional requirements of the human body are not the same for everyone since we all have a different genetic makeup that requires specific nutritional care. For one individual, they can eat a salad and feel satisfied, whereas another can eat an entire meal and still feel hungry. This is due to varying metabolic rates. So it's good to take a hard look at what you're putting in your body as the day progresses.

- Would your normal eating pattern qualify as 'healthy?'
- How much water do you drink in a day? How often do you reach for a soda or juice when you're thirsty?

- How much caffeine do you consume?
- Do you pay attention to your servings for each food group to make sure you're getting enough of the right types? How much of your meals consist of protein?
- Do you have access to freshly grown fruits and vegetables?
- Do you use supplements to make up for lack of vitamins or minerals in your diet?

Socializing

As countries have initiated lockdown protocols, our social lives took a hit to such an extent that we have had to learn the hard way how to be alone, or with the same group of people everyday. Here it is important to make time for reaching out to others to a certain extent where it is beneficial for you emotionally as well as for them. If there are people you find yourself constantly worrying about such as your parents, grandparents, elderly neighbor, or childhood friends.

Give yourself an emotional break by reaching out to these people in whatever safe way works best for both of you. Call your grandparents and just ask about their day, talk for 10 minutes, or however long you have. Drop a letter in your neighbors mailbox checking in, ask them if they would like to be your faux pen pal, even if you're right next door. Even if your relatives or neighbor are not receptive to this, reaching out and telling them you appreciate them is the smallest token that makes the biggest impact. You have time, what else are you doing after your work is done?

Physical Fitness

There is a certain stigma associated with rigorous and frequent exercise. Some people believe they need to force themselves to exercise until they are on the verge of collapse, to reach some unattainable beauty standard or to make a visible change in their health. This is not true. Based on your height, weight and dietary habits, an exercise program can be created to suit your needs and goals. As a general rule you should move your body or be active at least 30 minutes a day. You can take a walk, go for a jog, or run at your local track, as long as you can feel your heart rate increase and sweat. Some questions that you can ask to help yourself or find motivation are:

- Do you try to be active at least once a day?
- Do you prefer exercising alone or in a group?
- What goals do you want to have achieved by the end of this time?
- What safe spaces exist around your community where you are able to exercise?

The four pillars above take into question our basic needs, ensuring that we have effective coping mechanisms in place to live holistically during uncertain times. With that being said, the next method delves into the emotional aspect of COVID-19, and teaches us ways to really deal with a wide range of feelings and emotions. The good thing about emotions is that they are usually temporary, as the saying goes, "This too shall pass." With emotion-based coping strategies, you are going to be able to match your actions to your feelings, and start to realize why you react to certain situations like you do.

Dealing with Emotions

When you begin to feel sad, despondent, or that you are falling into a spiral of misery, it is best to work slowly and focus on soothing actions to better cope.

- Try cleaning a space in your house that has been overlooked while listening to music you like that is calming and soothing. This could be meditative ambient sounds, spoken word poetry, or an orchestra. It's up to you
- Make yourself a hot cup of tea and sit under a blanket with your favorite book.
- Practice yoga or breathwork for clarity and inner relaxation.
- Call a loved one and talk with them to feel grounded. You don't have to talk about your problems, but it is better for wellness if you let it out.

Many people's first instinct is to become angry, frustrated, or anxious in situations where there are no definitive answers. COVID-19 has provided so many possibilities for the outcome of society, and with most of the information provided by the government and elected leaders that we may feel will lead us astray this instinct to react with anger makes sense. Naturally, people are bound to feel frustrated, especially if their freedom of movement has been restricted, and they are only being told what to not do. If you feel this way there are some things you can do to move out of this emotion.

Try going for a walk, exercising, or making a clay model and smashing it! This specific form of anger management has shown to be extremely effective in releasing tension. You can play your favorite songs on blast and dance around your room to let it out. If you find a specific person or situation to be anger-inducing, write down what is making you angry, then rip the photo or letter into tiny pieces. This physical act demonstrates to your mind that you have the authority over each situation in your life, and you don't have to allow one specific situation to define your outlook on life.

Some people feel that dealing with their emotions is impossible, and that's why the options above are typically coupled with grounding practices. When we find ourselves in situations that provoke an intense emotional pain, finding your center allows you to focus on reality and what's in front of you. This practice can be mental or physical, and it typically involves describing the environment you are in using your five senses. For example, you can say that you hear the chirping birds outside, that you feel the softness of the t-shirt you are wearing, or you can smell the fruit trees outside. Another way to ground yourself is by playing a game. For example, choose a category and list all of the objects that fall under that category; like fruit: bananas, grapes, apples, oranges. Lists are a great way to focus while your mind makes sense of your current mental distress.

With physical grounding there is an intense focus on the touch of a small object. It can be a rock, a ring, or a piece of fabric, and this sensation allows you to change the immediate environment so a new sense of 'normal' can be achieved. This can also be done by running cold or warm water over the skin. Grounding should take from 20 to 30 minutes and be practiced regularly so reactions to anxiety and stress can diminish with time.

Another method of dealing with the stress of COVID-19 is by focusing on the breath and breathing deep. This is also referred to as breathing from your diaphragm, and is typically used in a wide variety of practices (spiritual, medical, even military) to improve your body's response to heightened levels of anxiety and stress. The effects that these emotions have on your body is targeted in your central nervous system resulting in a fight, flight, or freeze response. These responses wear down your body in many ways. Someone who feels on edge in this way for any extended period will find they experience shortness of breath, increased heart rate, dizziness, trembling, or sweating.

Practicing Mindfulness

Mindfulness is the final method that we will cover to manage our emotions during the pandemic. This concept is overlooked or misunderstood by most, and it means maintaining a moment-by-moment awareness of our thoughts, feelings, bodily sensations, and surrounding environment through a gentle, nurturing lens. Mindfulness allows us to remain grounded in stressful times, calming the inner storms that are distracting us from getting the most out of our lives.

Mindfulness also involves acceptance, meaning that we pay attention to our thoughts and feelings without judging them—without believing there's a "right" or "wrong" answer to how we are feeling in any given moment. When we practice mindfulness, our thoughts tune into what we are sensing in the present moment rather than reliving experiences from the past or imagining what could potentially happen in the future. Ultimately, mindfulness focuses on the now, not what has or will happen.

With roots in Buddhist meditation, this secular practice of mindfulness has entered the American mainstream in recent years, in part through the work of Jon Kabat-Zinn and his Mindfulness-Based Stress Reduction (MBSR) program, which he launched at the University of Massachusetts Medical School in 1979. Since that time, thousands of studies have documented the physical and mental health benefits of mindfulness in general and MBSR in particular, inspiring countless programs to adapt the MBSR model for prisons, schools and even certain healthcare institutions.

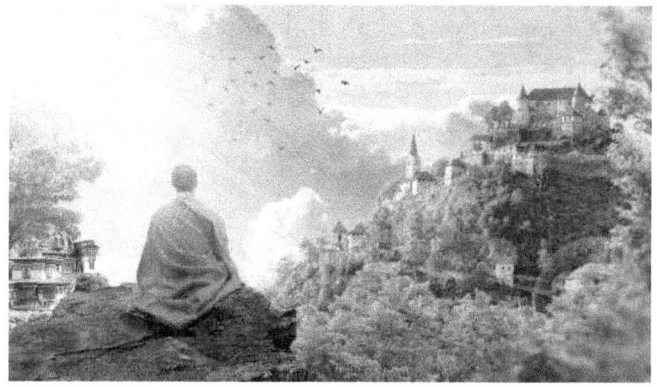

Studies have shown that practicing mindfulness, even for just a few weeks, can bring a variety of physical, psychological, and social benefits. Jon Kabat-Zinn emphasizes that although mindfulness can be cultivated through formal meditation, that's not the only way. It's not really about sitting in the full lotus, pretending you're a statue in a British museum. Mindfulness is about living your life as if it really mattered, moment by moment by moment by moment. A few key principles that you should take into consideration when performing mindfulness exercises, are the following:

- Pay close attention to your breathing, especially when you are feeling a very intense set of emotions. A few examples of these emotions include fear, anxiety, nervousness and even confusion.

- Be cognizant of what you are sensing in a given moment. Ensure that you are focusing solely on the sights, sounds, and smells that are often overlooked as you go about your day. This allows you to integrate with your surroundings, while establishing a newfound sense of calm.

- It is important to realize that your emotions do not define you. Remember who is in control, and that there is always a way to get out of a negative spiral of thoughts.
- Find "micro-moments" of mindfulness throughout the day. Use this as a way to refocus your day, maximizing productivity, and realigning your sense of purpose.

Mindfulness is not a method that always shows results, especially in the beginning. It requires time to refine and truly ascertain what methods of mindfulness are best for you. To help you better identify which method might work for you, here are a few options:

- Mindful breathing is seen in many different forms of meditation. It is during this process of breathing that there is a direct sense towards physical sensations, focussing on the air's passage both inside and outside of your body.

- The body scan practice focuses on the different parts of your body in a sequential manner. Typically, one starts from the head and ends at the toes, allowing you to holistically sense everything that is happening in your body, part by part.
- Walking meditation is a core focus on the movement of your body as you take each step. What you focus on is the feelings associated with your feet as they touch and leave the ground. What this form of mindfulness does is it allows us to realize actions that we take for granted, such as being able to walk.

Conclusion

The COVID-19 pandemic has influenced each and everyone one of us, some more than others. Our everyday life in its own way has become a barrier to the progression of society. Many have felt debilitated and helpless, while others have felt empowered by this time of isolation and motivated to work on themselves as better people. solve social

With vaccination still in testing phases across the world, the World Health Organization has done its best to implement preventative and protective measures to safeguard each person. Social distancing, regular washing of hands, as well as wearing a mask at all times has now become the norm. COVID-19 has served as a reminder that the life we live is so short and that we should take nothing for granted.

COVID-19 has had an even bigger reach than just the personal lives of the population, establishing itself within many different business domains. However, not all effects of COVID-19 have proven to be negative. The telecommunication, streaming, gaming and e-commerce industries have seen record highs, reinforcing our reliance on technology that is current, innovative and secure. We have seen how many countries panicked when COVID-19 reached their borders, not knowing how to control the virus. With lockdown restrictions being implemented across the globe, it is no surprise that many individuals feel cooped up, and have developed cabin fever. It is because of the impact of the technological industry, that the social spheres of our lives can still exist to shake up the monotony.

The effects of COVID-19 are broad and have established set challenges that need quick and reliable expertise to be effectively overcome. With officials struggling to find, isolate, and treat cases, and medical professionals working night and day we saw people's fears heightened. Luckily this has led to a conversation about America's flawed healthcare system that has been all but overlooked.

Local businesses began to close down due to a drop off in sales while tech companies saw an increase as those stuck at home looked for new ways to stay busy. Social gatherings were all but eliminated, and we all had to find new ways to connect with our loved ones. There were minimal avenues to express their hobbies and interests with gyms, movie theaters, sports clubs, and pool houses all being forced to close.

Luckily, the COVID-19 pandemic has influenced our adaptability and flexibility as humans and a collective culture. Although society as we know it has come to a standstill because of COVID-19, all hope is not lost. If anything, this pandemic has taught us that there are so many alternatives to express your passion and even make money off of them. To an extent it has made us realize who the important people are in our lives, and the person we want to see when we look in the mirror. Someday when we overcome this time in our lives, finally get past the stress of the pandemic and look back, we will be able to see what has changed us for the better. I hope the information obtained in this book has aided you in making more informed decisions, and you are able to estable a positive mindset towards COVID-19 pandemic.

References

Aten, J. (2020, April 2). *7 Ways to Cope With COVID-19*. Psychology Today. https://www.psychologytoday.com/za/blog/hope-resilience/202004/7-ways-cope-covid-19

Bary, E. (2020, October 30). *Visa and Mastercard have a lot in common, but COVID-19 puts one key difference in focus*. MarketWatch. https://www.marketwatch.com/story/visa-and-mastercard-have-a-lot-in-common-but-covid-19-puts-one-key-difference-in-focus-11604090026

BBC News. (2020, August 5). TV watching and online streaming surge during lockdown. *BBC News*. https://www.bbc.com/news/entertainment-arts-53637305#:~:text=Lockdown%20measures%20enforced%20due%20to

Carney, L. (2016, October 31). *Definitive Guide - How Much Should A Website Cost You? (Nov 19)*. Website Builder Expert. https://www.websitebuilderexpert.com/building-websites/how-much-should-a-website-cost/

Centers for Disease Control and Prevention. (2020, December 8). *CDC Library: COVID-19 Science Update: 12/8/2020*. Www.Cdc.Gov. https://www.cdc.gov/library/covid19/120820_covidupdate.html

Dixit, N., & McKee, J. (2020, May 21). *Paypal Well-Positioned To Gain Share In COVID-Related Digital Payments Shift*. Www.Spglobal.com. https://www.spglobal.com/marketintelligence/en/news-insights/blog/paypal-well-positioned-to-gain-share-in-covid-related-digital-payments-shift

Eugenio, S. (2017, February 9). *8 Cognitive Benefits of Playing Video Games for Kids*. Engadget. https://www.engadget.com/2017-02-09-8-

cognitive-benefits-of-playing-video-games-for-kids.html

Ferreira, N. (2019, June 6). *20 Advantages and Disadvantages of Ecommerce*. Oberlo. https://www.oberlo.co.za/blog/20-ecommerce-advantages-and-disadvantages

Igoe, M. (2020, December 7). *Biden's plan for global COVID-19 leadership to face early tests*. Devex. https://www.devex.com/news/biden-s-plan-for-global-covid-19-leadership-to-face-early-tests-98693

Institute of Medicine (US) Forum on Microbial Threats. (2007). Learning from Pandemics Past. In *www.ncbi.nlm.nih.gov*. National Academies Press (US). https://www.ncbi.nlm.nih.gov/books/NBK54171/

Intermountain Healthcare. (2020, April 2). *What's the difference between a pandemic, an epidemic, endemic, and an outbreak?*

Intermountainhealthcare.org. https://intermountainhealthcare.org/blogs/topics/live-well/2020/04/whats-the-difference-between-a-pandemic-an-epidemic-endemic-and-an-outbreak/

John Hopkins University, Faculty of Medicine. (2019). *2019 Novel Coronavirus: Myth vs. Fact*. John Hopkins. https://www.hopkinsmedicine.org/health/conditions-and-diseases/coronavirus/2019-novel-coronavirus-myth-versus-fact

MacIntyre, C. R., Seale, H., Dung, T. C., Hien, N. T., Nga, P. T., Chughtai, A. A., Rahman, B., Dwyer, D. E., & Wang, Q. (2015). A cluster randomised trial of cloth masks compared with medical masks in healthcare workers. *BMJ Open*, 5(4), e006577. https://doi.org/10.1136/bmjopen-2014-006577

Madhav, N., Oppenheim, B., Gallivan, M., Rubin, E., & Wolfe, N. (2017). Pandemics: Risks, Impacts, and Mitigation. *Nih.Gov*.

https://doi.org/10.1596/978-1-4648-0527-1/pt5.ch17

Sardona, J. (2017, November 19). *20 branches of science and their meaning - Brainly.ph.* Brainly.Ph. https://brainly.ph/question/1078052

Saxena, A. (2020, November 11). *How American Express is navigating the COVID-19 pandemic.* YourStory.com. https://yourstory.com/2020/11/money-matters-american-express-navigating-covid-crisis

Seladi-Schulman, J. (2020, April 24). *What's the Difference Between Viral and Bacterial Infections?* Healthline. https://www.healthline.com/health/bacterial-vs-viral-infections#diagnoses

Semuels, A. (2020, July 28). *Many Companies Won't Survive the Pandemic. Amazon Will Emerge Stronger Than Ever.* Time.

https://time.com/5870826/amazon-coronavirus-jeff-bezos-congress/

Sherman, N. (2020, June 2). Zoom sees sales boom amid pandemic. *BBC News*. https://www.bbc.com/news/business-52884782

Shwartz, M. (2019). *Biological warfare: an emerging threat in the 21st century: 1/01*. Stanford.Edu. https://news.stanford.edu/pr/01/bioterror117.html

Solís-Lemus, J. A., Costar, E., Doorly, D., Kerrigan, E. C., Kennedy, C. H., Tait, F., Niederer, S., Vincent, P. E., & Williams, S. E. (2020). A simulated single ventilator/dual patient ventilation strategy for acute respiratory distress syndrome during the COVID-19 pandemic. *Royal Society Open Science*, *7*(8), 200585. https://doi.org/10.1098/rsos.200585

Stevens, A. (2020). Governments cannot just 'follow the science' on COVID-19. *Nature Human Behaviour*, *4*(6), 560–560. https://doi.org/10.1038/s41562-020-0894-x

The Johns Hopkins Center for Health Security. (2020, August 19). *Interim Framework for COVID-19 Vaccine Allocation & Distribution in US*. Johns Hopkins Center for Health Security. https://www.centerforhealthsecurity.org/our-work/publications/interim-framework-for-covid-19-vaccine-allocation-and-distribution-in-the-us

Unity Technologies. (2020). *Eloqua - Error Information*. Img06.En25.com. https://img06.en25.com/Web/Unity/%7B1d8bb073-24ca-45ae-9b26-4ec9ac2e3fb4%7D_Unity-Monetization-Covid-19-Insights-v3.7.pdf?elqTrackId=0cf1b3ba3dd04d708e2731e75ddaa324&elqaid=2721&elqat=2

Vidyasagar, A. (2019, April 25). *What Are Bacteria?* Live Science; Live Science. https://www.livescience.com/51641-bacteria.html

World Health Organization. (2020). *Social Stigma associated with COVID-19.* https://www.who.int/docs/default-source/coronaviruse/covid19-stigma-guide.pdf#:~:text=The%20level%20of%20stigma%20associated

Image References

All images have been obtained by Pixabay

www.ingramcontent.com/pod-product-compliance
Lightning Source LLC
Chambersburg PA
CBHW070634220526
45466CB00001B/167